Endorsements

"Dr. Sauvage has prepared the *most comprehensive yet understandable book* for the education of *patients* with vascular disease *that I have ever seen.* It contains a wealth of information that is beautifully illustrated and presented with the upbeat, common-sense approach for which he is so well known. Because of this book, Dr. Sauvage will attain the *fondest hope* of every medical author -- that is, to help patients he will never meet, in places he will never visit."

- Norman R. Hertzer, MD
Chairman, Department of Vascular Surgery
The Cleveland Clinic Foundation, Cleveland, Ohio

"Just take 70 seconds and read the five cardinal rules for heart-healthy living (pages 184-187) and add five to ten high quality years to your life. *What a bargain!"*

- Peter Gloviczki, MD
Professor of Surgery
Division of Vascular Surgery, Mayo Clinic, Rochester, Minnesota

"I am enthusiastic about this book! Dr. Sauvage has done a remarkable job of condensing an immense amount of anatomy, physiology, pathology, surgery, medicine, nutrition, and psychology -- and even a touch of ethics -- into such a small and easily read volume. It is replete with illustrations that are lucid and to the point.

"This book could serve as an excellent source of good information for any layman interested in cardiovascular disease. More importantly, it is exactly what patients need to help them understand what their doctors tell them. This book will be of inestimable value to great numbers of patients whose doctors don't have the time to get their well-intentioned but often inadequate explanations across to them. *You Can Beat Heart Disease* will go a long way to help patients overcome fear and become successful, active, informed participants in their own care.

"I am pleased to give this book my highest recommendation."

- Wiley F. Barker, MD
Professor of Surgery
Division of Vascular Surgery
UCLA School of Medicine, Los Angeles, California

"*This is a gem of a book.* Clearly written and profusely illustrated, it sustains an easy and informative approach, in terms that can be well understood by those for whom it is intended, the many women and men from all walks of life who stand at risk of serious heart disease. And this is done without over-simplification or loss of accuracy. A consistent theme is that of prevention with sensible, practical, and effective recommendations for a heart-healthy lifestyle.

"*All Americans should read this book,* not only to learn more about themselves as marvelously complex living beings, but especially *to learn how easy it could be* to significantly reduce the immense burden of heart disease that is borne by modern society. Dr. Sauvage and his team should be complimented on this carefully crafted, clear, and articulate account of the greatest threat to human health we face today in the United States, and what steps we should take to control it."

- **David M. Robinson, PhD**
Director, Vascular Research Program
National Institutes of Health
National Heart, Lung, and Blood Institute, Bethesda, Maryland

"*This is a remarkable book.* Though written for laymen, a physician may take rewarding interest in reading it, too. It will help him brush up on his communication skills with his patients.

"The book describes in flowing and lively language understandable to any intelligent non-medical reader the anatomy, physiology, pathology, and therapeutics of the diseases of the heart and arteries. *There is not a question I can think of that a patient might ask for which this book does not provide an answer.*

"Two features struck me as particularly noteworthy. First, there is a profusion of simple but accurate line drawings to illustrate every detail suitable for pictorial representation. Perhaps even more impressively, the last chapter is a seldom seen, extraordinary summary of the spiritual values of what used to be called the art of healing. In this cynical modern world, putting such sentiments on paper is an act of great moral courage. The last lines reprint the *Prayer of St. Francis,* perhaps the tenderest summation of what human goodness is."

- **D. Emerick Szilagyi, MD**
Emeritus Chairman, Department of Surgery, Henry Ford Hospital, Detroit
Emeritus Professor of Surgery, University of Michigan School of Medicine
Founding Editor, *Journal of Vascular Surgery*

"Dr. Lester Sauvage is one of the pioneers of heart surgery. Yet he is more than a pioneering surgeon; he is a *visionary physician* who addresses not only the causes and prevention of heart disease, but also the soul of his patients."

- **Dean Ornish, MD**
Author, *Dean Ornish's Program for Reversing Heart Disease*
President & Director, Preventive Medicine Research Institute
Clinical Professor of Medicine
School of Medicine, University of California, San Francisco

"Upon opening this book you will be more than surprised. In a pocket-sized volume of some 300 pages you will find virtually everything you need to know about heart-healthy living, the background of modern cardiology, and the prevention and treatment of cardiovascular disease. And there's more. This fund of information is presented in such a clear manner that the most inexperienced and unsophisticated reader can understand it.

"Almost every page is specifically and instructively illustrated, and every topic is simply and concisely described. As I thumbed through this book before settling back to read it carefully, I wondered whether Dr. Sauvage would get to the subject of stents, or pacemakers, or a glossary, but no sooner had these ideas occurred to me than I came across these very subjects. And even more.

"Dr. Sauvage's extraordinary devotion to people shines through every page, exemplified by his citing of the Prayer of St. Francis which clearly enunciates his personal beliefs. Goodness of spirit shines forth like nothing I have seen before. I am not given to hyperbole, at least not easily, but in this case I can say that it is the *best book of its kind that I have ever read,* and I will cherish ownership of the final edition once it's in my hands."

- **Victor Parsonnet, MD**
Director of Surgical Research, Newark Beth Israel Medical Center
Clinical Professor of Surgery
New Jersey College of Medicine & Dentistry

"In *You Can Beat Heart Disease,* Dr. Lester Sauvage has provided an invaluable source of information to enlighten the layman about cardiovascular diseases. Beyond the informative and educational sections of this book that will appeal to all individuals, including medical personnel, Dr. Sauvage has provided a practical, common-sense approach to preventive measures. Additionally, he has provided valuable spiritual insight to help us contend with cardiovascular diseases. In my view, the goal of this book is to help us all live longer, happier, and healthier lives. Clearly, this goal has been accomplished."

- Calvin B. Ernst, MD
Professor of Surgery, Chief of Vascular Surgery Allegheny University of the Health Sciences of Philadelphia, Pennsylvania

"An *excellent book* for patients and their families. After reading it, I gave my copy to my parents so they could better understand atherosclerosis and how to prevent its impact on their health as they age."

- Julie Ann Freischlag, MD
Professor of Surgery
Medical College of Wisconsin, Milwaukee, Wisconsin

"Heart disease kills one out of every two American women -- yet this disease remains shrouded in confusion. Dr. Sauvage has performed a true feat by writing a straight-forward, understandable book that dispels much of the confusion and, because of this, will save many lives. Reading this book is a must for both heart patients and the general public."

- Nancy L. Snyderman, MD
Medical Correspondent, ABC News
New York, New York

Endorsements continued on pages 297-307.

cover design by Arthur Nakata
cover photo by Warren Berry

YOU CAN BEAT HEART DISEASE

*Vital information
to
help you live longer*

LESTER R. SAUVAGE, MD

with
Carol P. Garzona, Prevention Consultant,
Kathryn D. Barker, Medical Artist and Calligrapher,
and
Warren A. Berry, Director of Computer Graphics
& Medical Photography

THE HOPE HEART INSTITUTE

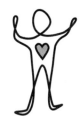

Better Life Press
Seattle, Washington

You Can Beat Heart Disease

Publisher's Cataloging-in-Publication Data
(Provided by Quality Books, Inc.)

Sauvage, Lester R., 1926-
    You can beat heart disease : vital information to help you live longer / Lester R. Sauvage ; with Carol P. Garzona, Kathryn D. Barker , and Warren A. Berry. -- 1st ed.
    p. cm.
    Includes index
    Preassigned LCCN: 98-70737
    ISBN 0-9663788-1-4

    1. Heart--Diseases--Treatment--Popular works.
    2. Atherosclerosis--Popular works.   I. Title

RD598.S28 1998   616.12
                                          QB198-422

TABLE OF CONTENTS

Foreword ix
Overview xiii
Dedication xv
Acknowledgments xvi

Strategy to Beat Heart Disease 1

Section I: **The Human Body:**
                 Its Systems and Its
                 Greatest Killer -- Hardening
                 of the Arteries (Atherosclerosis) 2-83

Section II: **Diagnosis** of the Two
                 Common Complications of
                 Atherosclerosis:
                    1. Blockage
                    2. Aneurysm Formation 84-111

Section III: **Prevention** of Atherosclerosis
                 and Its Complications by
                 How We Live Our Lives 112-181

Section IV: A Simplified Program for
                 Heart-Healthy Living 182-191

Section V: **Surgical Procedures** for Arteries
Irreversibly Damaged by
Atherosclerosis and Its
Complications 192-241

Section VI: **Related Heart Topics** 242-258

Section VII: **Spiritual Reflections** 259-262

Section VIII: **Glossary** * 263-282

Index 283-287

Review Questions to Help
You Help Others
Beat Heart Disease 288-290

Need for Research 291-293

**About the Author and
Team Members** 294-295

Message from Better Life Press 296

Endorsements
(Completion) 297-307

Concluding Thoughts 308

* **Some find it helps to review the Glossary first.**

Foreword

by

Jerry Goldstone, MD

This book is *about* each and every one of us, and it's for each and every one of us.

It's a book about our heart and blood vessels that examines the wonders of our anatomy, physiology, biochemistry, biophysics . . . and yes, even, spirituality.

No scientist or engineer could imagine being able to design, let alone build, so complex a pumping, distribution, and exchange system that could possibly work as efficiently and effectively as our cardiovascular system.

Most amazing of all, this system is expected to work flawlessly, without rest, for 80 to 100 years or more -- even when it's severely and repeatedly abused.

But like all complex systems, breakdowns and failures are inevitable, and as Dr. Sauvage and his team point out, cardiovascular disease is the leading cause of death in the United States, causing more deaths than cancer, accidents, and infections combined. Thus, it behooves us to learn more about cardiovascular disease so that its warning signs can be recognized and dealt with in order to prevent such problems as heart attacks, strokes, limb loss, and even death.

Another important reason to learn about the cardiovascular system is that dealing with diseases of the heart and blood vessels often requires choices to be made among and between various diagnostic tests, pharmaceutical agents, surgical procedures, and lifestyle changes. I believe it is important for each affected person to play an important role in making these choices. Fortunately, long gone are the days when physicians told patients "This is what you need," and the patients faithfully responded "Yes sir, you're the doctor."

Now, the choice is largely the patient's, while the physician's role is to provide information in order to help the patient make that choice. Unfortunately, more information is frequently needed or desired than many physician-patient consultations provide.

That is why this book, *You Can Beat Heart Disease,* is so important. It explains in clear and easily understandable words, illustrations, and x-rays what the cardiovascular system does, how it is made, how it works, what happens when it becomes diseased and doesn't work, and what can be done to fix it.

The book is based largely on the life-long experience of Dr. Lester Sauvage, a noted cardiovascular surgeon and research director, who spent 33 years repairing the hearts and blood vessels of thousands of grateful patients. What better way is there to gain understanding of the human cardiovascular system than to reconstruct it day in and day out? Who better understands the working of a Ferrari than a veteran Ferrari mechanic?

In spite of the fact that Dr. Sauvage is a surgeon, not all of the therapeutic options discussed in this book involve the traditional surgical maneuvers of cutting and sewing. The new, minimally invasive, catheter-based techniques are also appropriately described and discussed. Often the choice is between no operation or procedure, a catheter-based procedure, and a standard major operation. Aided by their doctors, well-informed patients are able to make these important decisions.

There is another lesson, perhaps even more important, to learn from this book. This lesson is that cardiovascular disease can be minimized and, in many cases, prevented by taking care of our bodies and minds by avoiding the things that we already know damage the heart and blood vessels: smoking, stress, and low-fiber diets high in saturated fat, *trans* fatty acids, sugar, and calories. We should also be doing more of the things that we know will lower our cardiovascular disease risk such as exercising regularly, eating a proper diet, and taking anti-platelet and anti-oxidant medications.

These preventive strategies are consistent with the well-known adage that an ounce of prevention is worth a pound of cure.

No health care system can treat and cure every illness. And this is where the responsibility clearly falls on the shoulders of each and every one of us. As individuals, and collectively as a society, it is up to us to take care of our cardiovascular systems, and we need to begin doing so at a young age to enable this complex system to run smoothly into old age at low medical cost.

Dr. Sauvage and his team have done us all a great service by providing so much valuable information in such a concise form. Now it's up to us to put this information to good use.

Jerry Goldstone, MD
Former Professor of Surgery
and
Chief of Vascular Surgery
University of California
School of Medicine
San Francisco, California

OVERVIEW
of this book,
and
its companion book,
The Open Heart

You Can Beat Heart Disease will take you on the journey of a lifetime through your body and its incredible heart and blood vessel system. Further, it will help you live a long and healthier life, while its companion book, ***The Open Heart,*** will help you find greater love and meaning in your extended years.

In *You Can Beat Heart Disease,* my team and I bring vital medical knowledge to you that could save your life. In *The Open Heart,* ten of my patients and I speak to you from our hearts about what matters most to us and how we have found the love which has continued to bring joy and meaning into each day of our lives.

In *You Can Beat Heart Disease* and *The Open Heart* you will find the information you need to defeat the Western world's greatest killer, heart disease, and to better appreciate each day of your life. *You Can Beat Heart Disease* will add years to your life, and the message of *The Open Heart* will make those years of living a true joy.

After reading *You Can Beat Heart Disease,* you will have a broad working knowledge of how your body functions. This information base will enable you to protect your arteries from becoming hardened and having clots form on their flow surfaces. Hardened arteries and clots cause heart attacks, strokes, high blood pressure, impaired walking, limb loss, and hemorrhage.

Preventing a disease is far better than treating it. Since how we live largely determines whether our arteries will remain healthy, we emphasize the individual's role in good health. *You Can Beat Heart Disease* tells you how to do this.

There is another reason why *You Can Beat Heart Disease* is important -- the rising cost of health care. The harsh economic reality is that our retired population is increasing rapidly and demanding high-tech medical care. This could mean bankruptcy for our nation early in the 21st century. It's simple arithmetic -- fewer people paying and more people receiving. Something has to give.

For the economic system of the United States to remain solvent as greater numbers of its citizens live longer, we must lower the total medical cost of keeping our older citizens healthy. *Each* of us has a responsibility to ourselves, our children, and our nation to make the lifestyle choices that will help us live as healthily as possible.

Our national goal must be to give the best care to all who need it. But for this to be economically feasible, we must decrease the number who require costly treatment. We ask all who read this book to help *others* make the lifestyle choices that will make this goal become a reality.

You Can Beat Heart Disease *can help you live a long and healthy life that will require a minimum of expensive medical care.* ***The Open Heart*** *can help you find increased joy in each day of your extended earthly journey.*

DEDICATION

This book is dedicated to the attainment of the wisdom and knowledge necessary to defeat the western world's greatest killers, *hardening of the arteries* and *clot formation.* Such a victory would lengthen life, decrease suffering, increase happiness, and, at the same time, reduce the high cost of medical care. These goals must be achieved because heart and artery disease due to these two conditions kills more people than cancer, accidents, and infections combined.

In this formidable effort to benefit humanity, all of us are inspired by the majesty of creation and by the peace and happiness of life when committed to helping others. We are awed by the universe, by our world, and especially by the zenith of God's creation -- the human being.

We recognize that one day we will all pass through the portal of death into eternity. But there is no reason to promote suffering and early death by living our lives in ways that will cause our arteries to become hardened, wear out at an early age, and fill with clot.

Instead, let us resolve to defeat heart and artery disease by how we choose to live. The importance of this choice is underscored by the fact that the majority of Americans choose poorly in this test for life. As a result, millions of our population will die prematurely of hardening of their arteries and clot formation. This book will help you live out the fullness of your years free of deadly heart and artery disease.

ACKNOWLEDGMENTS

I am deeply grateful to the following people for their invaluable contributions that have made this book possible:

Carol Alto for flawlessly transcribing the manuscript innumerable times and always being totally pleasant no matter the time nor the volume of work. In addition, her creative ideas have helped shape entire sections of the book.

Austine Fleming for her dedicated administrative work that enabled me to have the time to both direct the extensive research programs of The Hope Heart Institute and write the text of *You Can Beat Heart Disease.*

Mary Ann Harvey, Medical Editor of The Hope Heart Institute, for editorial and grammatical guidance.

Josh Rosenfeld of the Institute's Department of Clinical Research for searching out and verifying many of the obscure but incredible facts about our amazing bodies that are in this book.

Jeffrey D. Robinson, MD and **Philip J. Vogelzand, MD,** of the Department of Radiology of the Providence Seattle Medical Center for advice on radiologic matters.

Peter A. Demopulos, MD; **Milton T. English, MD**; **Bert Green, MD**; **C. Gordon Hale, MD**; **Tom R. Hornsten, MD**; **Peter B. Mansfield, MD**; **Michael Martin, MD**; **Gary E. Oppenheim, MD**; and **David C. Warth, MD,** of the Providence Seattle Heart Center for up-to-date details of current cardiology and endovascular coronary surgery.

Michael Zammit, MD, of the Providence Seattle Vascular Center for up-to-date details of peripheral vascular surgery.

Reneé Belfor, **Susie Wang**, and **Alison Evert** of the Nutrition Department of the Providence Seattle Medical Center for advice on dietary matters.

Keith Fujioka and his staff of the Pacific Vascular Laboratory at the Providence Seattle Medical Center for advice on ultrasound matters.

Dick Delson for important advice and invaluable editing of the manuscript.

Stan Emert for invaluable work at every level in all phases of this project, including developing effective plans to bring this book and its companion book, *The Open Heart (Updated Edition): Secret to Happiness,* to the widest possible audience.

Arthur Nakata for designing a cover that precisely captures the spirit of this book.

My family for their devoted support and encouragement throughout this endeavor, **especially my dear wife,** for her invaluable advice concerning all aspects of this project and to our **son John** for his essential help in making this book reader-friendly.

To **Jerry Goldstone, MD**, for writing the Foreword and to the many others who have endorsed this book, we are deeply grateful. They are:

Wiley F. Barker, MD

John J. Bergan, MD

Bradford C. Berk, MD, PhD

Nicholas J. Bez

Denton A. Cooley, MD

Herbert Dardik, MD

R. Clement Darling III, MD

Mr. Aires A.B. Barros D'Sa, MD

Calvin B. Ernst, MD

Thomas J. Fogarty, MD

Julie Ann Freischlag, MD

Peter Gloviczki, MD

H. Leon Greene, MD

Howard P. Greisler, MD

C. Rollins Hanlon, MD

Norman R. Hertzer, MD

Glenn C. Hunter, MD

Anthony M. Imparato, MD

Kaj H. Johansen, MD, PhD

J. Ward Kennedy, MD

John F. (Jack) Kiley

John W. Kirklin, MD

Robert L. Kistner, MD

Floyd D. Loop, MD

John A. Mannick, MD

S. A. Mellick, CBE, MD

Yasutsugu Nakagawa, MD

Lloyd M. Nyhus, MD

John Ochsner, MD

Dean Ornish, MD

Victor Parsonnet, MD

Malay Patel, MD

Malcolm O. Perry, MD

Joseph C. Piscatella

Charles Rob, MD

Francis Robicsek, MD, PhD

David M. Robinson, PhD

Robert B. Rutherford, MD

Stephen M. Schwartz, MD, PhD

Nancy L. Snyderman, MD

Ronald J. Stoney, MD

D. Emerick Szilagyi, MD

Jesse E. Thompson, MD

Frank J. Veith, MD

J. Leonel Villavicencio, MD

Vallee L. Willman, MD

James S.T. Yao, MD, PhD

Christopher K. Zarins, MD

SPECIAL
ACKNOWLEDGMENT

For 33 years of my life, I had the good fortune to practice medicine at the **Providence Seattle Medical Center.** From that experience, I can say that there is no better place to receive kind, loving care in an atmosphere of scientific excellence.

It's easy for the human touch to be lost in the medical practice of today. Yet, the care at the Providence Seattle Medical Center encourages me. Its dedicated staff still has concern for all -- including the poor and the vulnerable.

Strategy
to
Beat Heart Disease

In this book we present ....

general **concepts**,

specific **information**,

and clear **directions**

.... that will help you beat heart disease

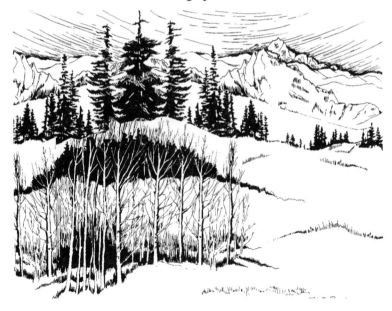

... Perspectives ...

Section I:
The Human Body

Its Systems and Its Greatest Killer -- Hardening of the Arteries (Atherosclerosis)

Introduction 4-7
The Cell 8-11
The Life Cycle 12-15

The 11 Major Body Systems 16-39
    1. Musculoskeletal System 18
    2. Nervous System 19
    3. Cardiovascular System,
       an Overview 20-21
    4. Hematopoietic (Blood Cell
       Forming) System 22-23
    5. Lymphatic/Immune System 24-25
    6. Respiratory System 26-27
    7. Digestive System 28-29
    8. Urinary System 30-33
    9. Endocrine System 34-35
    10. Reproductive System 36-37
    11. Integumentary (Skin) System 38-39

Boundary Organ Concept 40-43

The Cardiovascular System,
    a Detailed Examination 44-83

Three Main Parts 44
   1. **Power Source**, the Heart 45-54
     • Circulatory Cycle and
       Color Changes
       of Blood 46-47
      • Tireless Worker 48
      • Four Chambers 48
      • Four Valves 48-49
      • Diastole and Systole 50-51
      • Two Coronary Arteries 52-53
      • Congestive Heart Failure 54-55

   2. **Conduit System**, the Blood Vessels 56-63
      • Arteries 56-58
      • Capillaries 59
      • Veins 60-63

   3. **Transport Medium**, the Blood 64-67

Blood Clotting and Embolus
  Formation 68-71

Atherosclerosis -- the Most
  Frequent Abnormality that
  Affects Our Arteries 72-83
    General Considerations 72-76
    Two Main Complications 77-83
      1. **Blockage** of Flow Channel 78-79
        Nature's Attempt to
         Compensate 80-81
      2. **Aneurysm** Formation 82-83

Introduction

Few assets are more valuable than good health, a precious gift we seldom fully appreciate until we lose it.

In the pages ahead you will learn how to keep your heart and blood vessels healthy. This book will be a joyful adventure in learning how to live a long, healthy, and happy life, free of the ravages of arterial disease that cause heart attacks, strokes, high blood pressure (of kidney origin), impaired walking, amputations, and hemorrhages.

We will explain how the most common disease in the Western world -- *hardening of the arteries* -- causes many arteries to *block off* and lesser numbers to *blow out.* We will tell you how to prevent this from happening. But if preventive measures have been started too late or have been ineffective, we will show you how damaged arteries can be repaired or replaced by surgery.

When the blood levels of cholesterol and fats are high, these lipids invade the inner portion of the arterial wall and cause plaques to form. Bone-like calcific deposits occur around some of these plaques and make the wall hard. This hardness gives the condition its popular name, *hardening of the arteries.* The *medical term* for this condition is *atherosclerosis.*

Hard plaques may thicken the arterial wall, narrow the flow channel to some degree, and make the flow surface rough and ulcerated. Not all plaques are hard. Some remain soft, and most of these are small.

Oily, gruel-like, fatty material may form in the center of the soft plaques. This lipid core is often covered over by a dangerously thin cap of fibrous tissue which is prone to rupture. If this happens, the greasy material contained in the core drains into the flow channel where it can cause the blood to clot (a process whereby fluid blood becomes like soft "Jell-O"). Should the cap of a soft plaque in a coronary artery of your heart rupture, you could die. This is the most common cause of heart attacks. Though less frequent, heart attacks are also caused by clots which form on the diseased flow surface of hard plaques.

In some people, atherosclerosis affects the arteries differently, especially the aorta (the biggest artery). Instead of *blocking* the flow channel, atherosclerosis weakens the aortic wall so much that the blood pressure stretches it and forms thin-walled enlargements called *aneurysms* which may rupture (blow out) and cause fatal hemorrhage.

Nearly 45% of all deaths in the industrialized world are caused by blocked arteries and aneurysms due to atherosclerosis. This staggering total is 50% greater than the number of deaths due to all types of cancer. In fact, it is greater than the number of people who die from cancer, accidents, and infections *combined.*

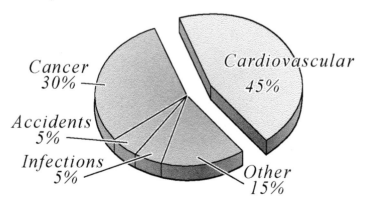

Figure 1 - Causes of death in the United States.

But before you become pessimistic about the ominous threat of *atherosclerosis* and *clot formation* which causes 95% of the deaths due to heart and artery disease in the western world, there is good news to tell. Proper application of the preventive measures described in this book could prevent up to 90% of these premature deaths. These preventive measures could also save your lungs from emphysema, prevent many cancers, and keep you from developing diabetes.

If preventive measures are applied too late or prove inadequate, there is still hope since most arteries damaged by atherosclerosis and clots or by aneurysm formation can be repaired or replaced surgically. Even so, patients undergoing surgery must take the best of care of themselves for the rest of their lives to obtain optimal results. This is so because surgery is only a mechanical solution to a structural problem. Surgery does nothing to correct the underlying biochemical abnormalities that cause the inner part of the arterial wall to harden and clots to form on its flow surface.

Our primary goal in this book is to help you keep your arteries free of blockages and blowouts so you will remain healthy, or become so if you aren't now, live a long life, and avoid a lot of medical expense.

To assist you in doing this, we will first consider three subjects that will help you to better understand your body. These subjects are the *cell,* the *life cycle,* and the organization of the body into *11 major organ systems.* **We consider this broad base of knowledge essential for you to develop a heart-and-spirit-healthy life style that will enable you to take charge of your health.**

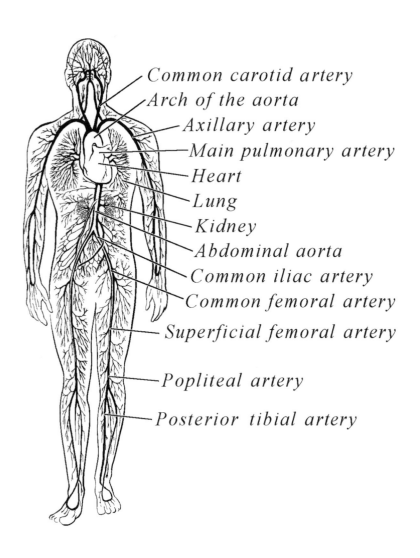

Common carotid artery
Arch of the aorta
Axillary artery
Main pulmonary artery
Heart
Lung
Kidney
Abdominal aorta
Common iliac artery
Common femoral artery
Superficial femoral artery
Popliteal artery
Posterior tibial artery

"The Lifelines Within Us" -- Our Arteries

The Cell

Cells are the smallest organized units of life. They are the building blocks from which all tissues and organs are formed. Cells float in a clear water-like liquid called interstitial fluid. Each cell is a unique world unto itself. About 100 trillion (100,000,000,000,000) cells form our adult physical structure.

Oxygen fuels the chemical reactions required for cells to perform their complex functions. Nerve cells discharge electric impulses. Muscle cells contract. Stomach cells secrete digestive juices. Each type of cell has its own special function.

The outer border of the cell is formed by a membrane composed largely of phospholipids, a special type of fat. This fatty composition makes the membrane insoluble in water and enables it to contain the watery contents of the cell. The membrane's other essential job is to selectively regulate what goes in and out of the cell. Oxygen, water, nutrients, and other chemicals go in, while carbon dioxide and other waste products come out.

The inside of the cell is formed of a soft, semi-fluid "Jell-O"-like material called *cytoplasm*. Located throughout the cytoplasm are many structures including those called *ribosomes* that make proteins, and others called *mitochondria* which produce the energy required by the cell.

A round body in the central part of the cell, called the nucleus, is formed of even more specialized "Jell-O"-like material which is also surrounded by a fatty membrane. Within the nucleus there are about 100,000 specialized collections of the chemical regulators of life, the **DNA** (**d**eoxyrib**o**nucleic **a**cid) molecules, called *genes*.

Genes are DNA molecules that start, direct, and stop life. They are grouped into specific aggregates called *chromosomes*.

Some Different Cell Types

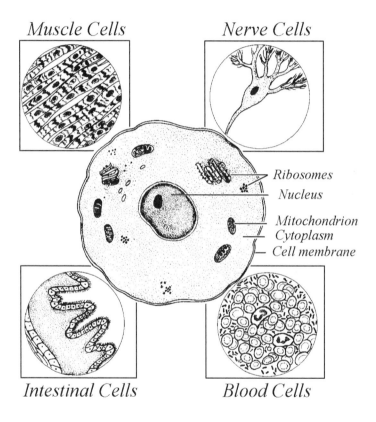

Muscle Cells

Nerve Cells

Ribosomes
Nucleus
Mitochondrion
Cytoplasm
Cell membrane

Intestinal Cells

Blood Cells

Figure 2 - Schematic representation of a "typical" cell and of various cell types. Only four of the many different structures inside the "typical" cell are shown.

The nucleus of every cell of our body has 46 chromosomes, except for the ovum of the female and the sperm of the male, which have 23. The DNA of each gene sends a chemical messenger called **RNA** (**ribo**nucleic **a**cid) into the cytoplasm to direct the ribosomes to manufacture one specific protein.

Through its RNA messengers, the DNA of the genes directs the manufacture of all the body's proteins, whether for function, growth, or replacement of worn-out parts. Proteins form the enzymes which direct the manufacture of fats and carbohydrates.

DNA is also responsible for the perpetuation of life itself by giving the ovum and the sperm the ability to unite and reproduce the species.

Each cell that forms must be nourished by the blood which the heart pumps through the circulatory system.

We will discuss the arteries, capillaries, and veins that make up this system in detail later (pages 56-63). For now, we will simply say that the systemic arteries carry red blood away from the left side of the heart and deliver it to the tiny blood vessels called capillaries which wind in and out of the minute spaces between the body's innumerable cells.

Oxygen, water, nutrients, and other chemicals in the blood pass through the thin walls of the capillaries into the clear fluid in which the cells float. From there, these life-sustaining materials diffuse into the cells. Waste products, including carbon dioxide, diffuse from the cells in a reverse sequence into the blood, now blue, at the far end of the capillaries. From here, the blood flows on into the systemic veins which return it to the right side of the heart.

Capillaries

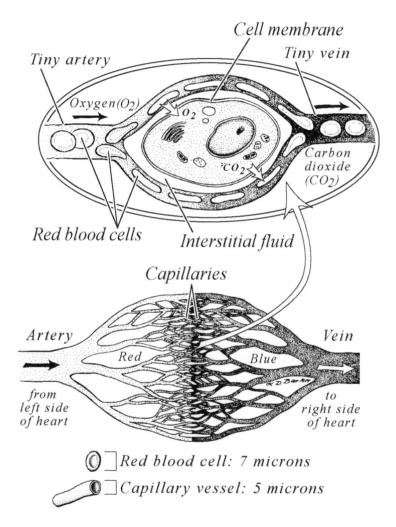

Figure 3 - Capillary blood nourishes the cells and removes waste products from them. Red blood cells are bigger than the capillary vessels and must elongate to pass through them single file. The red blood becomes blue as it goes through the capillaries and gives oxygen to the cells.

The Life Cycle

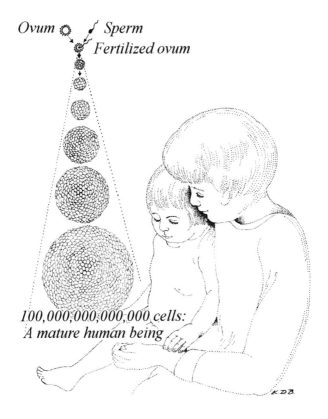

Ovum ○ ♂ Sperm
            Fertilized ovum

100,000,000,000,000 cells:
A mature human being

Figure 4 - Our life cycle is a mystery beyond compare . . . two cells unite to become one which divides to become two, and those two become four, and those four become eight, and those eight become sixteen, etc., etc., etc., to become a developing entity recognizable as human by four weeks with all the major organ systems taking form. The cells develop in different ways. Some become heart cells, others brain cells, still others bone cells, etc. The growth process continues in an infinitely precise and orderly manner, leading to the birth of a helpless human infant nine months after conception.

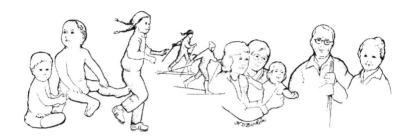

The Life Cycle

The human body is a wondrous result of human and divine creation. It arises from the union of the two generative cells . . . one male, the *sperm,* and one female, the *ovum* . . . to form one fertilized cell called the *zygote,* whose inception signals the beginning of a new human life. This fertilized cell attaches to the protective tissue of the inner wall of the uterus known as the "endometrium." There the miracle of creation continues for nine months through an absolutely incredible sequence of cell division and cell specialization into 11 major systems. Then the human infant is born, totally dependent on others for every care and necessity of life.

After birth, the infant's body continues to develop and grow as its cells multiply throughout infancy, childhood, and adolescence until the adult stage is reached at about 20 years. At that time the body weighs 20 to 25 times more than at birth and is composed of approximately 100,000,000,000,000 (100 trillion) cells. In terms of our planet's population, we have 20,000 *times* more cells in our body than there are people in the entire world. Yes, hard to believe . . . but true.

Water accounts for about 60% of our body's weight. A 200-pound man has about 120 pounds of water (14.2 gallons) in his body. About 10 pounds (1.2 gallons) are in his blood. About 30 pounds (3.6 gallons) are in the fluid in which his cells float. About 80 pounds (9.4 gallons) are in his cells.

Without water to drink, we would live only a few days. We're not as dependent on water as fish, but we come close.

Even more amazing than the development of our physical body is the development of our spiritual self that determines what kind of person we become. The proper development of the spiritual and emotional side of our lives requires that we receive *love* and *protection* in our early formative years.

Our brain is more complex and has greater ability than any computer man has ever built. If its emotional circuits are established early on for hate and rage instead of for love and peace, they will be very hard to change later.

Neglected and abused children often develop selfish and possessive circuitry in their brains that causes them to become unhappy adults, frequently with little sense either of justice or compassion. These deficiencies are the root cause of many of our nation's current social problems. In fact, the future of our country depends much more on the character and emotional state of the men and women our children become than on how much money they will make.

Our children's physical development is determined by heredity, diet, exercise, and the habits they develop. As parents we can't change the first factor, but we can change the others because we are responsible for every care in their early formative years. As our children grow and develop, our role becomes more and more one of providing direction and guidance to their lives by the *example* we set for them.

After we become adults, our physical condition depends largely on how we take care of ourselves. We can allow our bodies to become overweight and weak, or we can live our lives in a heart-healthy manner that will enable most of us to live enjoyably into advanced years at low medical expense.

Atherosclerosis is an accelerated wearing-out process that is mainly caused by the way we live. This process hardens the arteries of huge numbers of people in the United States and other industrialized nations, killing nearly half of those who die in these countries by blocking the flow channels of vital vessels or causing their walls to rupture.

But there is hope! Most people can prevent this hardening process from developing or, if present, from advancing, by choosing to live a heart-and-spirit-healthy life.

The prime purpose of this book is to assist you, your children, and grandchildren in this vital selection process.

By making the proper choices for a healthy life, most of us will reach advanced years in a vital manner, enjoying each day of our earthly journey as we do so.

But we need to recognize the obvious, as Dr. H. Leon Greene states on page 307, that "even a perfect lifestyle will not prevent the inevitable . . . we will all ultimately die." Accordingly, we should also prepare in our own time and way for this transition to eternity, remembering that it is the *connecting link to all that lies beyond.*

The 11 Major Body Systems

We are more than a mere mass of cells. We are so much more. We are human and possess profound physical, mental, and spiritual dimensions. Our physical components are a marvel of technical efficiency with control mechanisms far more exacting than those of any machine.

As humans, we begin at conception, grow, are born, continue to grow, mature, age, and eventually die. In this incredible journey we move, sleep, breathe, eat, drink, see, feel, hear, smell, taste, talk, maintain our temperature, digest our food, eliminate wastes, replace parts that wear out, heal injuries, and much, much more.

And our mental and spiritual dimensions are even more mysterious and grand. They enable us to love, make decisions, create, feel deeply, compose music, write poetry, record history, appreciate, forgive, see a divine purpose in our lives, and ever so much more. We are a marvel of creation, set apart from all else on earth. And how can all this be . . . from just two cells that become one?

In the formative days of our life before birth, the dividing cells of our developing structure differentiated into the innumerable cell types which then went on to form the 11 major systems of our bodies. We will now consider the broad outlines of these miracles of creation in the sequence listed below. Then we will devote special attention to the cardiovascular system in order to appreciate how it serves every one of the 100 trillion cells that comprise our mature physical being. **The 11 major body systems are:**

1. Musculoskeletal System
2. Nervous System
3. Cardiovascular System
4. Hematopoietic (Blood Cell Forming) System
5. Lymphatic/Immune System
6. Respiratory System
7. Digestive System
8. Urinary System
9. Endocrine System
10. Reproductive System
11. Integumentary (Skin) System

We believe that understanding the structure and function of the human body will help all of us live a heart-healthy life. The most practical way to gain this knowledge is to consider the essence of these 11 systems of the body.

1. The Musculoskeletal System

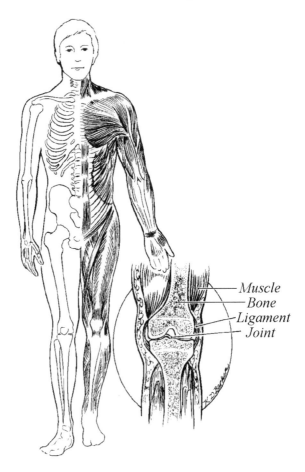

Figure 5 - The musculoskeletal system provides us with form and, in concert with the nervous system, the ability to move. Bones interconnect with other bones through movable connections known as "joints." Muscles arise from a bone on one side of a joint and attach to the bone forming the other side of the joint. When these muscles are stimulated to contract (shorten) by the nervous system, our bones and joints move and this motion enables us to walk, run, jump, and dance.

2. The Nervous System

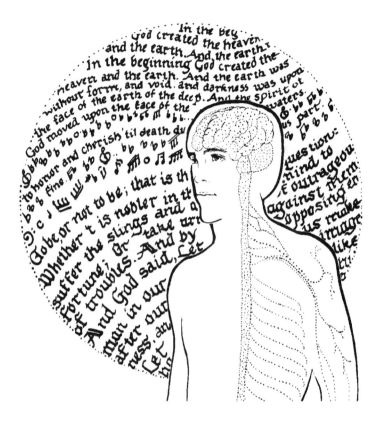

Figure 6 - The nervous system, composed of the brain, spinal cord, and nerves, provides us with the ability to feel, move, balance, see, hear, smell, think, remember, and much more. But of all our wonderful human capacities, our emotional and intellectual capabilities are the most mysterious, such as our capacity to say "I love you," feel compassion, know right from wrong, admit error, ask for forgiveness, write books, identify problems, provide solutions, invent machines, play music, have a sense of destiny, pray, and seek a close relationship with our God.

3. The Cardiovascular System
- an overview -

The cardiovascular system has three main parts:
1. A **heart** that pumps 40 million times a year.
2. A vast network of **vessels** that, if placed end-to-end, would form a tube approximately 60,000 miles long.
3. The **blood** that fills the system.

There are two sets of three types of vessels -- arteries, capillaries, and veins -- that interconnect through the right and left sides of the heart to form a continuous figure-eight circulatory pathway. One set of vessels, called the pulmonary circuit, carries blue blood to the lungs and red blood from the lungs. The other set of vessels, called the systemic circuit, carries red blood to the cells and blue blood from the cells.

Arteries start out big at the heart, give off branches, and become progressively smaller. Capillaries are tiny; they nourish the cells. Veins start out small, join together, and get progressively bigger as they get closer to the heart.

Arteries carry blood away from the heart to the capillaries; veins carry blood from the capillaries back to the heart.

The majesty of the human body is symbolized by the vastness of the blood vessel system through which the right side of the heart pumps the blue blood to the lungs and the left side of the heart pumps red blood to the cells of the body. The red blood supplies all the cells with the oxygen, water, nutrients, and other chemicals they need to survive and function while the blue blood removes carbon dioxide and other waste products from the cells.

This amazing system is presented in detail on pages 44-83.

Arteries of the Body

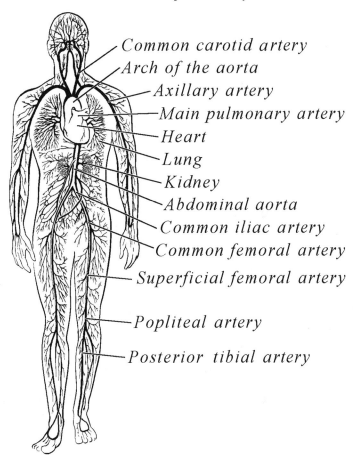

- Common carotid artery
- Arch of the aorta
- Axillary artery
- Main pulmonary artery
- Heart
- Lung
- Kidney
- Abdominal aorta
- Common iliac artery
- Common femoral artery
- Superficial femoral artery
- Popliteal artery
- Posterior tibial artery

Figure 7 - The arterial system. The right side of the heart receives the oxygen-depleted blue blood returning through the systemic veins (not shown) from the body, and pumps it through the pulmonary arteries to the capillaries of the lungs where it takes up oxygen, gives off carbon dioxide, and again becomes red. The left side of the heart receives this red blood returning through the pulmonary veins (not shown) from the lungs and pumps it through the systemic arteries to the capillaries of the body where it gives oxygen to and removes carbon dioxide from the cells and again becomes blue.

4. The Hematopoietic
(Blood Cell Forming) System

The hematopoietic system produces the cells and cell fragments found in blood. These include the *red* blood cells that carry oxygen; the *white* blood cells (granulocytes*, lymphocytes, and monocytes) that protect us from infections and cancer; and the *platelets* (tiny pinched-off portions of a big bone marrow cell) that stop bleeding and promote healing. These cells and the platelets are formed in the honeycomb-like tissue called *bone marrow* that fills the inside of our bones.

The life span of a red blood cell is about four months, a granulocyte about six hours, different types of lymphocytes from a few days to many years, and a platelet about 10 days. About 2-1/2 million red blood cells, one million white blood cells, and 1-1/2 million platelets wear out each second and are replaced by an equal number of new ones. And there are many other such balances in our bodies.

For a moment consider that even if Ford, Chrysler, and General Motors were combined, they could not make one car per second. This is so, even though making a Cadillac car is less complex than making a red blood cell.

Blood is composed of about 40% cells and 60% fluid. Most of the cells are red, while a small percentage are white. The fluid, called *plasma,* contains special chemicals -- sodium, potassium, calcium, magnesium, oxygen, carbon dioxide, proteins, fats, carbohydrates, cholesterol, vitamins, enzymes, hormones, and many more. The beating heart powers the blood through the vessels so that it can nourish all the cells of the body with what they need to survive and function.

* **cyte = cell (from the Greek)**

The Hematopoietic
(Blood Cell Forming) System

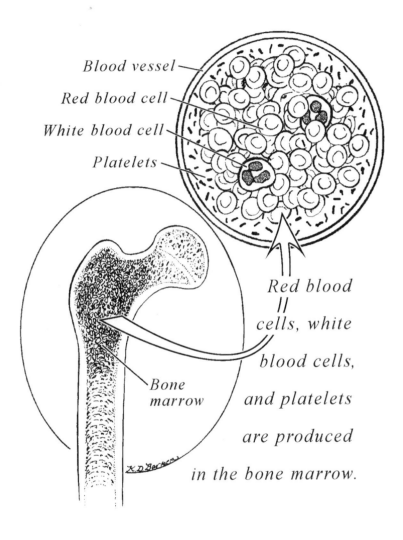

Blood vessel
Red blood cell
White blood cell
Platelets

Red blood
cells, white
blood cells,
and platelets
are produced
in the bone marrow.

Bone marrow

Figure 8 - The red blood cells, white blood cells (granulocytes, lymphocytes, and monocytes), and platelets are formed inside our bones in the honeycomb-like tissue called bone marrow.

5. The Lymphatic/Immune System

The lymphatic system consists of thin-walled *lymph channels*, interspersed collections of lymphatic tissue *(lymph nodes)*, clear fluid called *lymph* (filtered out from the blood) that flows slowly through this system, and *lymphocytes* (cells that circulate in the blood and lymph). The lymph returns to the blood through a big lymph channel which joins a large vein at the base of the neck on the left side. **The lymph system has three important functions:** first, to *protect* us from chronic infections and cancers; second, to continuously *refresh* the fluid that the tissue cells float in; and third, to *transport* digested fat from the bowel to the blood.

The immune system consists of the *lymphatic system, spleen*, and *thymus.* These three components protect the body from bacteria, viruses, fungi, and cancer cells. The spleen is about the size of an open hand and is located in the upper left portion of the abdomen. The thymus is located in the upper front part of the chest directly behind the breast bone. It is very large in infancy, but shrinks with age, becoming largely replaced by fat in the adult.

Some lymphocytes make special proteins called *antibodies* that attack bacteria, viruses, fungi, and cancer cells. These proteins circulate in the blood where they lock onto the surface of these invaders and kill them. Most importantly, these lymphocytes continue to make these protein weapons for long periods, sometimes permanently. For example, the vaccine for smallpox is composed of a weak virus that causes only a mild reaction. But this mild reaction gives the vaccinated person permanent immunity from ever being infected with the strong virus that causes the severe disease.

The Lymphatic/Immune System

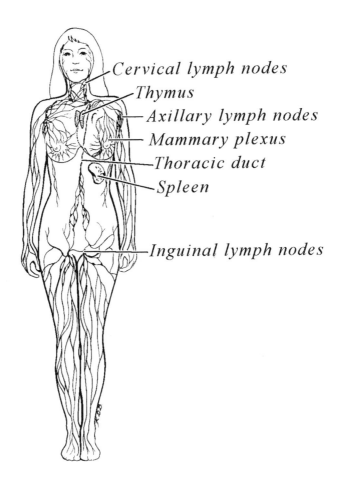

Cervical lymph nodes
Thymus
Axillary lymph nodes
Mammary plexus
Thoracic duct
Spleen

Inguinal lymph nodes

Figure 9 - The lymphatic/immune system is a vital defense mechanism for our body. Loss of even a portion of it -- as occurs in advanced AIDS -- is usually fatal within a year or two from infections with bacteria, fungi, and viruses, and often from the development of cancer, as well.

6. The Respiratory System

The respiratory system is composed of *three parts*: an upper, a middle, and a lower airway. This system has two main functions: first, to provide oxygen to and remove carbon dioxide from the blood; and second, in concert with the nervous system, to enable us to speak.

The *upper airway* consists of the nose and pharynx. The *middle airway* consists of the larynx (voice box) and the trachea (windpipe) and its two divisions (right and left main bronchi), and in turn, their major subdivisions. The *lower airway* (lungs) consists of increasingly smaller air passages which branch into approximately 600,000,000 tiny one-cell thick air sacs (alveoli) that have a combined surface area of about 2,000 square feet. These air sacs are covered on their outer surfaces by tiny blood vessels (*capillaries*) that, too, are but one cell thick. Oxygen passes in and carbon dioxide passes out through these walls.

The oxygen content of the air in the alveoli is higher than the oxygen content of the blue blood in the capillaries, while the carbon dioxide content of this blood is higher than that of the air in these tiny sacs. When we breathe in, oxygen diffuses from the air sacs into the blue blood and turns it red, while carbon dioxide diffuses from the blood into the air sacs. The exchange of these gases enables the circulating blood to carry *oxygen to* and *remove carbon dioxide* from all the cells of the body.

The incredible balance of nature is exquisitely shown in the way plants and animals use air. Animals use oxygen and make carbon dioxide in the oxidative chemistry of living, while plants use carbon dioxide and make oxygen in the photosynthetic chemistry that enables them, and us, to live.

The Respiratory System

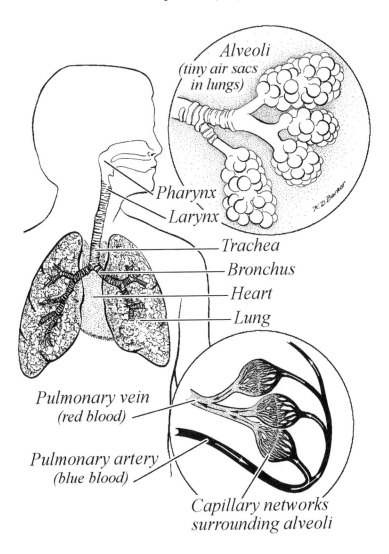

Figure 10 - This system is constructed to provide a massive surface for interface of the oxygen-depleted blue blood (returning from the body) with the atmosphere. In this reaction, the blood surrounding the tiny air sacs takes up oxygen to become red and gives off carbon dioxide.

7. The Digestive System

The digestive system is a continuous tube about 40 feet long that passes in a semi-meandering way throughout the core portion of our bodies, beginning at the mouth and ending at the anus. This system functions as a "conveyor belt" that is loaded with supplies (food) and fluid (water) at the mouth, where the digestive process begins by chewing and swallowing. The ingested food and water are moved slowly along the "conveyor belt" by a massaging, undulating forward motion of the "belt" known as *peristalsis.* The food is digested into ever smaller chemical units as it moves from the mouth into the esophagus and on through the stomach into the bowel.

When the food has been broken down into its component chemical sub-units (complex carbohydrates into simple sugars, proteins into amino acids, and fats into fatty acids) by the action of the powerful digestive enzymes secreted by the glands in the mouth, stomach, pancreas, duodenum, and small intestines (bowel), these sub-units are absorbed into the blood and lymph (which transports the digested fat into the blood). Laden with these products, the blood flows to the liver where processing occurs to form compounds that the body needs. The liver, weighing about four pounds, is the giant chemical factory of the digestive system, in fact, of the entire body.

Our liver excretes a greenish fluid called *bile* that contains cholesterol. This fluid flows out through the bile ducts. The gall bladder, an out-pouching of the main bile duct, stores bile and, after we eat, empties it into the duodenum to assist in the digestion of food. Some components of the bile are reabsorbed into the blood, taken to the liver, and reprocessed.

The peristaltic action of the intestines continues to move the indigestible portions of our food (along with excess water, bile, matter excreted by the intestinal glands, cells shed from the surface of the bowel, and friendly bacteria) through the small bowel (jejunum and ileum) into the large bowel (colon and rectum), and finally through the anus to the outside of the body as a "bowel movement."

The Digestive System

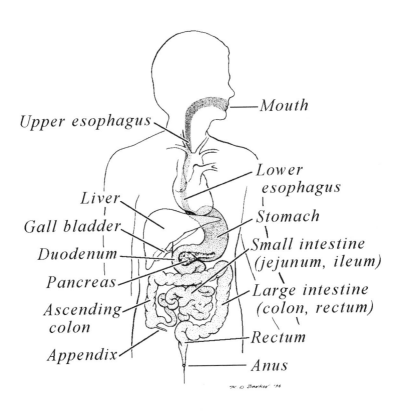

Figure 11 - The digestive system provides a vast surface upon which our food is broken down into its basic components that are absorbed into the blood and lymph and carried to the liver for further chemical processing.

8. The Urinary System
(With Comments About the Artificial Kidney and Kidney Transplantation)

The urinary system is composed of two kidneys, each connected by a drainage tube *(ureter)* to the bladder where a single drainage tube *(urethra)* empties to the outside of the body.

The kidneys have about 90 miles of fine tubules that are masterpieces of filtration and chemical efficiency. These tubules remove waste products, excess water, and extra minerals from the blood; selectively concentrate them; and then excrete what's left as a yellow fluid called *urine*.

If the kidneys stop functioning, death usually occurs within a few days due to toxic elevations of potassium in the blood that cause the heart to stop. Should the kidneys fail, their function can be taken over by a machine that "washes" the blood or by an exchange method that puts fluid into the abdomen and removes it a few hours later. These methods enable large numbers of patients with no function of their own kidneys to live for many more years.

If a suitable donor kidney for transplantation becomes available and the patient's condition is satisfactory, a transplant may be possible. Unfortunately, this logical solution to a very large medical problem is inadequate because there are many more patients in permanent kidney failure who require chronic treatment with the artificial kidney for continued life than there are donor kidneys that are suitable for transplantation. There are over 10,000 kidney transplants done each year in the United States. The need is far greater.

The Urinary System

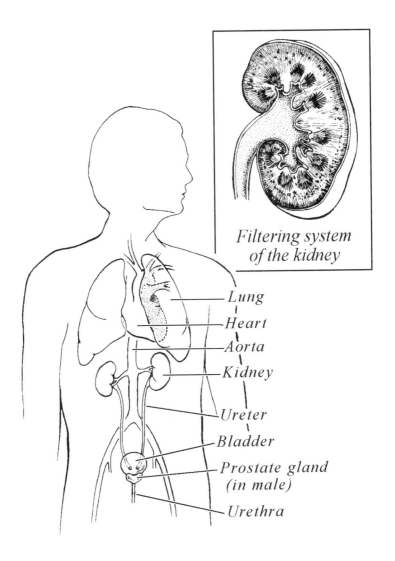

Filtering system
of the kidney

Lung
Heart
Aorta
Kidney
Ureter
Bladder
Prostate gland
(in male)
Urethra

Figure 12 - To keep the water content and chemistry of the blood in balance, the kidneys filter about one quart of blood each minute.

In the U.S. today, nearly 200,000 patients with chronic kidney failure are able to live reasonably normal lives because of the artificial kidney. These patients, who would otherwise die within days, are attached to an artificial kidney three times a week for periods of three to four hours. During that time about 2/3 of a pint of their blood is run through the machine per minute, removing waste products, excess water, and minerals from it. This "washing" of the blood is called *hemodialysis*.

The connections to the machine are established by placing two large needles into a vein in the forearm, one to bring the patient's blood to the machine which "washes" it and the other to return the "washed blood" back to the patient. The bigger this vein and the stronger its wall, the better it can function for dialysis.

The best way to develop such a vein is to make a direct surgical opening between an adjacent artery and vein near the wrist. The blood in the high pressure artery rushes through this opening into the low pressure vein and causes it to become enlarged and thick-walled all the way up the forearm.

These changes in the vein are essential if it is to be used successfully for hemodialysis treatments three times a week over a long period of time. During the first year alone, the vein must be punctured by big needles at least 312 times.

But if a suitable direct connection can't be made between an adjacent artery and vein, it may be possible to place an artificial blood vessel graft between an artery in one part of the forearm and a vein in another part. In this instance, the needles are placed into the artificial graft.

When possible, the direct connection of an artery to a vein is preferred for hemodialysis access because such a vein will usually function for a much longer time before closing off than will an artificial graft.

Some patients can't use hemodialysis because they have no suitable veins that can be punctured to establish connections with the kidney machine. For these patients, a procedure called *continuous ambulatory peritoneal dialysis* can be used instead. An advantage of this technique is that the patients can be up-and-about while the dialysis is taking place in the abdomen.

In this method, 2 to 3 quarts of a dialysis fluid are run through a special connector into the peritoneal cavity (the space in the abdomen that contains the stomach, bowels, and liver) where it is left for several hours and then drained out. More fluid is added. The cycle is repeated 3 to 4 times a day. The fluid is replaced at bedtime, left in overnight, and drained out in the morning. This repetitive cycle is continued day-in, day-out.

During the time the fluid is in the peritoneal cavity, waste products, excess water, and extra minerals diffuse into it and are removed when the fluid is drained out. Though somewhat less efficient than hemodialysis, peritoneal dialysis is preferred by many patients who wish to self-administer their treatment at home because the peritoneal method is easier for them to learn and carry out.

The dramatic evolution of the science of treating kidney failure has led to the medical specialty of *nephrology* and to the surgical specialties of *hemodialysis* and *kidney transplant surgery*. Today, few people die of kidney failure in the developed countries of the world.

9. The Endocrine System

The endocrine system is made up of a series of glands (pituitary, thyroid, parathyroid, islet cells of the pancreas, adrenals, testicles in males, and ovaries in females) that make special chemicals called *hormones* which are secreted directly into the bloodstream where they circulate to distant organs and influence their function in vital ways.

For example, the *pituitary gland* is called the "master" gland of the body, because it secretes hormones that control the function of the other endocrine glands. It also secretes a hormone that controls growth and another that enables the kidneys to reabsorb needed water from the filtration tubules. Without this latter hormone, we would die from loss of water within a few hours.

The *thyroid gland* secretes a hormone called *thyroxine* which regulates the metabolic rate of our bodies. This hormone determines how fast our "motor" runs.

The *parathyroid gland* secretes a hormone called *parathormone* that controls the calcium content of our body, which in turn influences the beat of the heart, the contraction of muscles, and the structure of bones.

One type of *islet cell* of the *pancreas* secretes a hormone called *insulin* (absent, reduced, or ineffective in diabetics) which enables our cells to use glucose (sugar) for energy and, when there's an excess, to store it as glycogen in liver and muscle cells. Another type of islet cell secretes a different hormone called *glucagon* which causes the glycogen to release glucose when more energy is needed.

The *adrenal glands* secrete several hormones; one of these, called *adrenaline,* enables us, in times of stress or danger, to get that instant acceleration we need to react beyond our usual capacity. Other adrenal hormones, such as *cortisone* and *aldosterone,* control much of the vital chemistry of life relating to stress, minerals, sugar, and water.

The *testicles* secrete "testosterone," and the *ovaries* secrete "estrogens" and "progesterone." These hormones make men and women different.

The Endocrine System

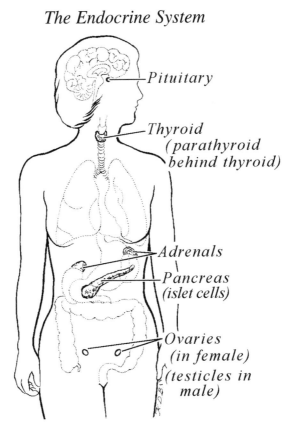

Figure 13 - The endocrine system controls the chemistry of our bodies. Without its hormones, we would die in minutes.

10. The Reproductive System

The reproductive system begins with a cell source (ovaries in the female for the ovum, and testicles in the male for the sperm) upon which the continuation of the human race depends.

The remainder of the reproductive anatomy in both the male and female is pertinent to the union of these two cells to form a fertilized ovum that develops within the uterus into that most remarkable of all earthly mysteries, the *human infant.*

The reproductive system has the dual purpose of continuing the human race and, in my personal belief, of being involved in the expression of mutual love between husband and wife.

The Reproductive System

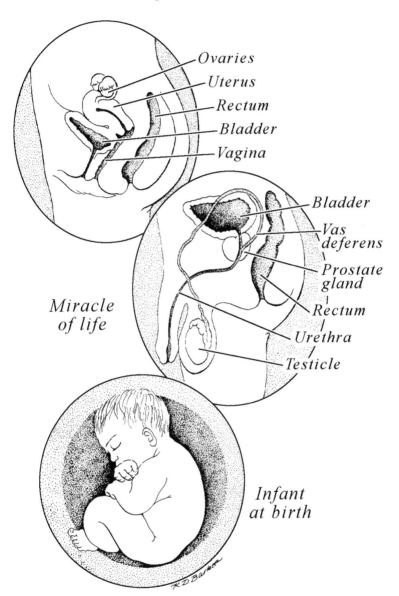

Ovaries
Uterus
Rectum
Bladder
Vagina

Bladder
Vas deferens
Prostate gland
Rectum
Urethra
Testicle

Miracle of life

Infant at birth

Figure 14 - The reproductive system is responsible for the continuation of human life on this planet.

11. The Integumentary (Skin) System

The integumentary system comprises the outer covering of our bodies, and so to speak, we live within it. Although few people think of the skin as an organ, it is actually the largest (and in many ways the most unusual) organ of the body. The average adult has about 16 square feet of skin, generally somewhat less for women than men.

The skin has **three vital functions:** first, to *keep* the underlying tissues from drying out (serving like the peel of an orange or the skin of an apple); second, to *prevent* bacteria, fungi, and viruses from invading our bodies; and third, to *maintain* our body temperature within a precise zone. To facilitate this latter function, the skin has approximately 2 million sweat glands. The skin is so important that if these functions are impaired or lost over a substantial portion of the body, as from a major burn, the patient may die despite the best medical care.

Heat is produced by the chemical reactions ongoing in each of our 100 trillion cells. Our body temperature is kept nearly constant at 98.6 degrees Fahrenheit (37 degrees Centigrade) so that our cells can function in an optimal manner. Maintenance of this critical balance is achieved by regulation of the amount of heat that is lost through the skin. This is accomplished by precise control of two complex functions: the volume of blood flowing through the deeper layer of the skin and the amount of sweat evaporating from the surface of the skin.

The greater the volume of blood flow through the skin, the greater will be the loss of heat from its surface, provided that the temperature outside the body is less than the temperature inside.

When the weather is hot and the generation of heat within the body is high, as during exercise, the sweat glands of the skin become active. As this sweat evaporates, the heat of vaporization is taken largely from the surface of the skin, cooling it (and the body) in the process.

The Integumentary (Skin) System

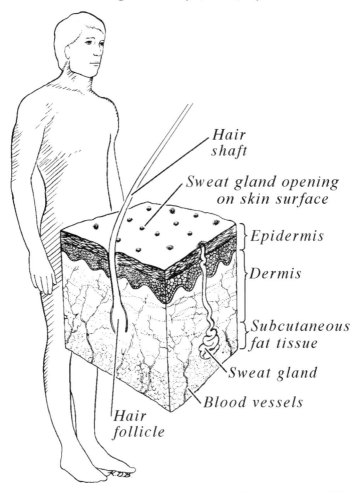

Figure 15 - This system protects us from the outside world and keeps our body temperature at 98.6 °F.

The "Boundary Organ" Concept

Let us now consider how the circulation of blood through our vessels, the *lifelines* within us, sustains the 100 trillion cells of our bodies by providing them vital contact with the outer environment through the lungs, intestines, liver, kidneys, and skin. In this broad context, these organs make up an exchange zone where oxygen, water, nutrients, and other chemicals are brought into the body, and carbon dioxide, other waste products, and heat are removed from it.

The needs of every cell of our bodies must be taken care of by these boundary organs. Blood is the vehicle that enables this vital commerce to occur.

What and how much we eat is critically important to this exchange. There are three basic food types: carbohydrates, fats, and proteins (please see glossary). In brief, carbohydrates (4 calories/gram) are used for energy; fats (9 calories/gram) are a vital component of every cell's walls and are also used for energy; and proteins (4 calories/gram) form the engines (muscles), regulators (enzymes), structures (tissue), and machinery (cell components) of our bodies.

Blood circulates through the lungs, intestinal tract, and liver to receive oxygen, water, nutrients, and other chemicals from the outside world. The blood then carries these supplies to the body's cells where they are utilized in the chemical reactions of life that generate energy and heat, repair damaged parts, and synthesize new compounds. The waste products of these reactions pass into the blood which delivers them to the lungs, liver, intestines, kidneys, and skin where they are discharged to the outside as components of breath, feces, urine, radiant energy and heat of vaporization (sweat).

The "Boundary Organ" Concept

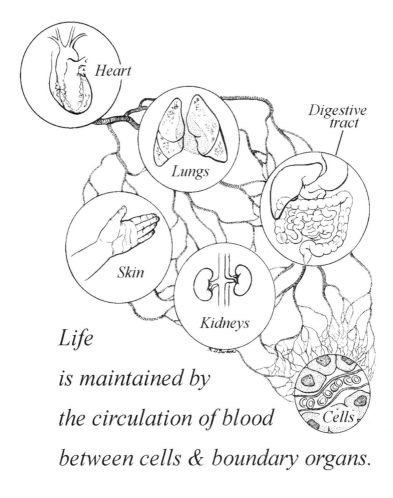

Life is maintained by the circulation of blood between cells & boundary organs.

Figure 16 - The boundary organ concept asserts that for the cells of the body to survive, they must all have contact with the outside world. The circulation does this by connecting the cells to the boundary organs where the exchange occurs. In this manner, the cells obtain what they need and discharge what they don't need.

The Lungs

In the lungs, respiratory gases are exchanged with the atmosphere. When we breathe in, fresh air fills the tiny air sacs of the lungs and enables oxygen to diffuse into the blue blood flowing through the capillaries that surround the alveoli. In these capillaries, oxygen combines with hemoglobin (the iron-containing-protein in the red blood cells) to form *oxyhemoglobin,* a bright red-colored compound, which turns the blue blood red. As this is happening, the blood releases carbon dioxide which diffuses into the air sacs. When we breathe out, this "stale" air with its load of carbon dioxide and decreased amount of oxygen is expelled from our lungs into the outside air.

Oxygen is needed to fuel the chemical reactions in each cell. These reactions produce carbon dioxide which would become harmful if high concentrations were to develop. This does not occur because the venous blood continuously transports carbon dioxide from the tissues to the lungs where the excess is exhaled to the outside world.

We breathe faster and more deeply during strenuous exercise to supply our muscles with the added oxygen they need and to remove the extra carbon dioxide they produce. Precise control mechanisms regulate these adjustments.

Our crucial dependence on a continuous supply of oxygen to our cells is shown by what would happen if our hearts were to stop suddenly. We would lose consciousness in about 10 seconds. In fact, we would be "out" before we hit the floor because our brain would go blank before our muscles would lose their tone and cause us to collapse. And by four minutes, many of our brain cells would be damaged beyond repair from lack of oxygen.

The Intestines

The intestines are like a grocery store where the cells of the body place their orders for food and water. In a real sense, they are at our mercy because their selection is limited to what we provide them by the diet we eat. What we force our arteries to consume may harden their walls and cause clots to form on the flow surface.

In the intestines, food is chemically broken down, combined with water, absorbed into the bloodstream and lymphatics, and carried to the liver for further processing. From there the blood flows to the lungs, and then on to the tissues to supply the needs of each cell for oxygen, water, nutrients, and other chemicals.

If totally deprived of water, we would die of dehydration in several days. If totally deprived of food, we would die of starvation in several weeks.

The Kidneys

Waste products are produced constantly in our cells and are carried by the blood to the kidneys, where most are excreted in the urine along with excess water and minerals to keep our body's chemistry in proper balance.

The Skin

The skin functions as a huge convection and vaporizing surface to release excess heat into the outer environment at a rate that will keep our body temperature nearly constant at 98.6° F (37° C). This precise temperature regulation is essential for the optimal function of the many enzymes that regulate the chemical reactions in our cells.

The Cardiovascular System
- a detailed examination -

Three Main Parts

The three main parts of the cardiovascular system are:
1. **Power source**
2. **Conduit system**
3. **Transport medium**

The *power source,* the **heart,** is an almost inexhaustible pump that beats over 100,000 times each day. No other muscle can do so much work. The *conduit system* is a huge network of **vessels** that if placed end-to-end would wrap twice around the earth at the equator and extend for an additional 10,000 miles. The *transport medium,* the **blood,** through the propulsive power of the heart and vast scope of the distribution system, reaches every one of the body's 100 trillion cells and supplies their needs.

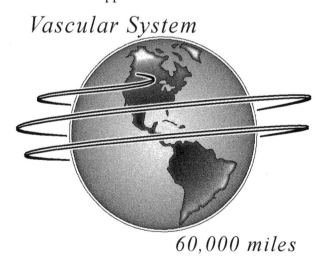

Vascular System

60,000 miles

Figure 17 - The blood vessels of one person if placed end-to-end would encircle the earth at the equator nearly 2-1/2 times.

1. Power Source -- The Heart

The heart is a muscle pump (with valves) that beats in a rhythmic manner to propel blood through an incredible system of vessels to supply the body's 100 trillion cells. Our life depends on the continuous flow of blood from heart to cells and back again in a never ending cycle.

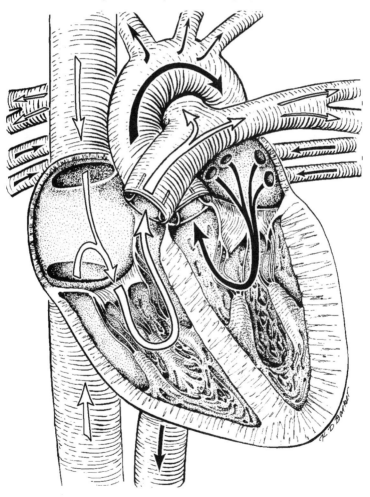

Figure 18 - The Human Heart.

Circulatory Cycle
and
Color Changes of Blood

The circulatory pathway of the blood is composed of a
figure-eight circuit with one loop (the systemic) for the body
and one loop (the pulmonary) for the lungs. Each loop has an
arterial and a venous component connected by a capillary
bed. The blood is blue in the systemic veins and pulmonary
arteries and red in the pulmonary veins and systemic arteries.

The right side of the heart receives the blue blood returning
through the systemic veins from the body and pumps it on
through the pulmonary arteries into the capillaries of the
lungs where it combines with oxygen and turns bright red.
This red blood flows on through the pulmonary veins into the
left side of the heart which pumps it forward through the
systemic arteries into the tiny capillaries that supply the 100
trillion cells of the body with oxygen. The color of the blood
turns "blue" as this happens. This blue blood flows back
through the systemic veins into the right side of the heart,
completing the circulatory cycle. If this cycle stops, we die.

The blue blood turns red in the capillaries of the lungs when
oxygen combines with the dark blue colored reduced
hemoglobin in the "red" blood cells to form the bright red
colored *oxyhemoglobin.* Then, after the arterial blood gives
up part of its oxygen to the cells, the blood becomes "blue"
again. The more oxygen the "red" cells give up to the tissues,
the darker (more blackish) these cells and the blood become.

Color Changes of Blood

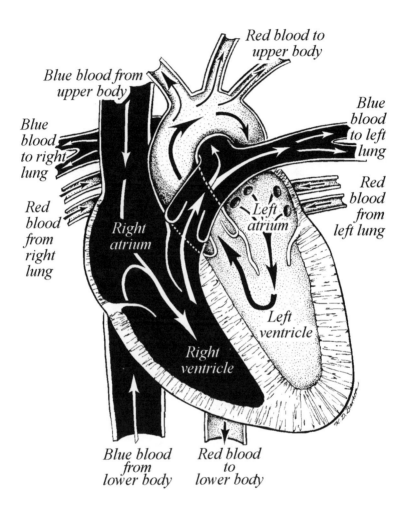

Figure 19 - Arrows indicate the circulatory pathways of the blue blood (shown as black) returning from the body to be pumped by the right side of the heart to the lungs and the circulatory pathways of the red blood (shown as stippled) returning from the lungs to be pumped by the left side of the heart to the 100 trillion cells that comprise our bodies.

Tireless Worker

The heart is the power source for life -- a blood pump that can never rest. The heart beats about 80 times/minute (faster during exercise and slower during sleep), 4,800 times/hour, 115,000 times/day, 40 million times/year, and one billion times in 25 years.

During maximal exercise the heart pumps up to four times what it does at rest, with most of the blood going to the working muscles. Even calculated on resting output alone, the adult heart pumps about 1-1/2 gallons of blood/minute, 90 gallons/hour, 2,200 gallons/day, 800,000 gallons/year, and 56 million gallons in 70 years (equal to what the mighty Amazon empties into the Atlantic in one second).

Four Chambers

On the right side, the heart has a receiving chamber (right atrium) to receive the blue blood returning from the tissues (depleted of oxygen and laden with carbon dioxide) and a pumping chamber (right ventricle) to pump it to the lungs. On the left side, the heart has a receiving chamber (left atrium) to receive the red blood returning from the lungs (replenished with oxygen and depleted of carbon dioxide) and a pumping chamber (left ventricle) to pump it back to the tissues to supply the cells.

Four Valves

The heart must have well-functioning valves to work efficiently: two inlet valves to open when the ventricles are ready to fill and two outlet valves to open when the ventricles are ready to eject. Thus, the heart has four valves, an inlet valve and an outlet valve for both the right and left ventricles. The inlet valves are the *tricuspid* on the right and the *mitral* on the left. The outlet valves are the *pulmonary* on the right and the *aortic* on the left. If these valves don't open or close properly, the heart muscle must do extra work to pump the volume of blood that is required to adequately nourish all the body's cells.

Valves of the Heart

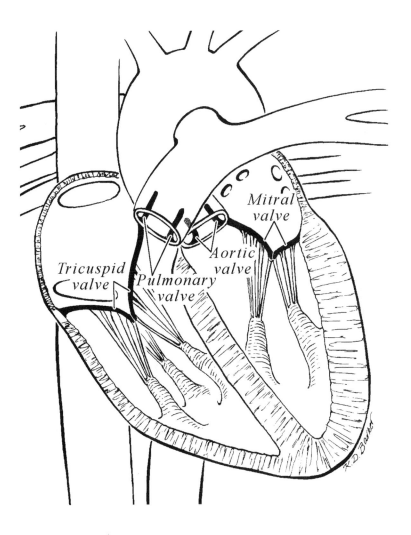

Figure 20 - Heart has four valves.

Diastole and Systole

Diastole is the blood-filling phase of the heart beat. The heart must fill before it can empty. In diastole the inlet valves (tricuspid and mitral) open as the outlet valves (pulmonary and aortic) close, allowing the blue blood from the body to flow into the right ventricle and the red blood from the lungs to flow into the left ventricle.

Heart in Diastole

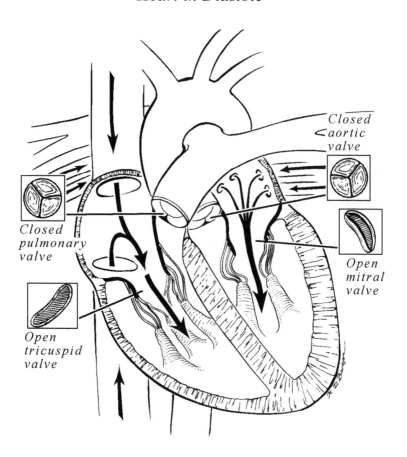

Figure 21 - Filling of ventricles in diastole.

Systole is the contracting or pumping phase of the heart beat. As the ventricles begin to contract, their inlet valves (tricuspid and mitral) close and shortly thereafter their outlet valves (pulmonary and aortic) open as the pressures in the respective ventricles rise above those in the pulmonary artery and aorta. The continuing contraction of the right ventricle pumps the blue blood to the lungs while that of the left ventricle pumps the red blood to the body.

Heart in Systole

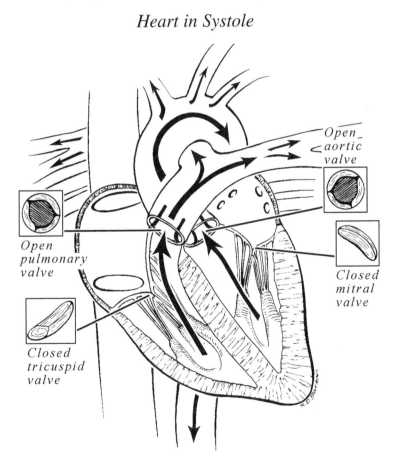

Figure 22 - Emptying of ventricles in systole.

Two Coronary Arteries
- The Heart's Fuel Lines -

For the heart muscle to do its work, it must be nourished by an adequate supply of well-oxygenated (red) blood. This "high octane fuel" reaches the muscle cells through two arteries, called the *right* and *left* coronaries.

The left coronary is about 1/4 inch in diameter where it originates from the aorta, while the right is usually a little smaller. These two arteries, the first branches of the aorta, receive about 5% of the blood that the heart puts out at rest.

The volume of blood that flows through the coronary arteries depends on our level of activity and varies from about 1/2 pint per minute at rest to 2 pints per minute at maximum exercise.

For the heart to do more work, it must receive more oxygen and nutrients. This means a greater supply of red blood. If the heart's entire blood supply were to be suddenly cut off, the heart would become weak and ineffective within a minute or two and would soon stop entirely.

The heart, which weighs only about 2/3 of a pound (roughly 0.4% of the body's weight), consumes about 10% of the oxygen used by the entire body, even though, when contracted, it's only about the size of your fist.

Both of the *coronaries* have two main branches, which in turn have branches, and these branches branch, etc. In developed, industrialized countries, blockage of the coronary arteries from atherosclerosis and clot formation kills nearly as many people as all other causes of death combined.

Coronary Arteries of the Heart

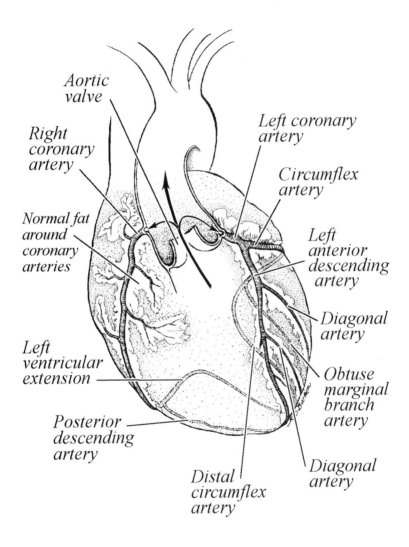

Figure 23 - Heart is nourished by two coronary arteries, a right and a left.

Congestive Heart Failure

When the heart fails, it can't pump enough blood to the cells of the body to enable them to function properly. The most frequent causes of this condition are decreased blood supply to the heart muscle due to coronary artery disease (atherosclerosis) and clot formation, reduced numbers of muscle cells as a result of heart attacks (due to coronary artery disease), impaired valve structure (causing either obstruction, leakage, or both), high blood pressure (hypertension), and viral infections of the muscle cells of the heart.

No matter the cause, heart failure makes the patient weak because the tissues don't receive enough oxygen and nutrients to do their work. If the left ventricle fails, the blood backs up into the lungs and causes them to fill with water. This forces the exhausted patient to fight for each breath. If the right ventricle also fails, the blood backs up into the brain, liver, kidneys, intestines, and legs, causing them to swell. Congestive heart failure is an agonizing way to die -- breathless, weak, confused, unable to eat, and compelled to sit up and gasp for air.

Fortunately, congestive heart failure can often be improved by medicines which cause the kidneys to excrete more salt and water, by diets that restrict salt intake, by drugs which increase the strength of the heart beat, and by agents that expand the small arteries and decrease the blood pressure. If heart failure is due to abnormal valve function or to lack of coronary blood supply, surgery to correct these problems may be very beneficial. But for patients with worn-out hearts, transplantation is their best chance for recovery. The problem is that there are many more patients dying of heart failure than there are donor hearts available for them.

Person in Congestive Heart Failure

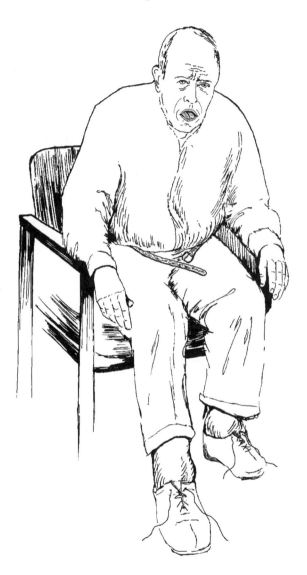

Figure 24 - This individual has failure of both the left and right sides of the heart. He is weak, gasping for breath, unable to lie down, and has swelling of his brain, liver, kidneys, intestines, and legs.

2. Conduit System -- The Vessels

We have three types of blood vessels -- arteries, capillaries, and veins. The structure of these vessels in the pulmonary and systemic circuits is similar, though the walls of the systemic arteries are thicker. The systemic arteries carry the red blood pumped by the left side of the heart to the tissue capillaries where it gives oxygen, water, nutrients, and other chemicals to the cells, and removes waste products from them. The systemic veins then return this blood, now blue, back to the right side of the heart which pumps it through the pulmonary arteries to the alveolar capillaries where it takes up oxygen, loses carbon dioxide, and turns red. This blood returns through the pulmonary veins to the left heart.

Systemic Arteries

Arteries are relatively thick-walled tubes made up of three different layers of tissue that surround a channel (lumen) through which the blood flows to the capillaries. From a functional standpoint, arteries connect the heart to all the cells of the body. They are indeed the *lifelines* within us.

The *innermost layer* is the thinnest and is called the intima. It's lined with delicate cells called *endothelium* which are in direct contact with the blood flowing through the lumen.

The *middle layer* is the thickest and is called the *media.* It is made up of alternating circular sequences of elastic fibers, smooth muscle cells, and collagen fibers.

The *outermost layer*, called the *adventitia*, is composed of loose fibrous tissue containing small blood vessels called the *vasa vasorum* (vessels of the vessels) that penetrate the outer portion of the media and nourish its cells.

The cells of the intima and the inner portion of the media to a depth of about 1/50 of an inch are nourished by diffusion of oxygen, water, nutrients, and other chemicals from the red blood flowing through the lumen. Beyond that depth the wall is nourished by the vasa vasorum. In veins, these tiny vessels extend much closer to the flow surface than they do in arteries.

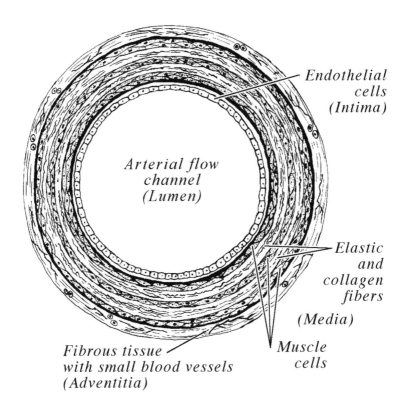

Figure 25 - Cross Section of a Systemic Artery.

When the heart contracts (systole), it pumps blood out into the aorta and its big branches. This surge of blood increases the blood pressure which causes the muscle cells and fibers of the media to elongate.

This elongation increases both the length and width of these big vessels, enabling them to hold more blood. In diastole the elastic recoil of these expanded components helps "pump" this blood to the tissues.

The combination of hardening of the arteries and clot formation is by far the most common cause of death in the industrialized world. If an artery becomes blocked as a consequence of this disease, the tissues that it nourished will likely die from lack of oxygen and nutrients.

The aorta, the biggest artery, is, in a sense, like the trunk of a tall tree. The trunk rises up from the roots (the heart) and has many branches. These branches branch and the branches in turn branch, becoming progressively smaller as they do so. The main trunk gets smaller as this branching occurs. At the level of the navel, the trunk divides into two large branches of equal size called the common iliac arteries; one of these vessels descends on each side to supply its half of the pelvis and the leg below.

The arteries branch until they are so tiny that they can only be seen with a high-power microscope. Then, they connect with the vast sea of still tinier vessels called *capillaries* that nourish the 100 trillion cells of the body.

No one knows why atherosclerosis develops frequently in all of the bigger arteries but rarely does so in some of the smaller ones, as the internal mammary arteries inside the front of the chest, and never develops in the tiny arteries.

Systemic Capillaries

The capillaries -- incredible in number and microscopic in size (one endothelial cell thick, and less than one-tenth the width of the finest human hair) -- receive the red blood from the arteries and form seemingly endless networks of tiny channels that surround the trillions of cells which make up our bodies. The combined surface area of all the capillaries is about 3,000 square feet, an area slightly larger than that of a tennis court. Each one of the billions of capillaries in our body nourishes hundreds of cells. Oxygen, water, nutrients, and other chemicals in the blood pass through the capillary walls into the clear liquid the cells float in and diffuse from there into the cells to supply their needs.

The waste products which arise from the chemical reactions of life that go on in each cell diffuse out into the fluid around the cells. From there, these products pass through the capillary walls into the blood of this vast network of lacy microvessels which merges into the tiny veins that are the beginning of the systemic venous system which returns the blood, now blue, back to the heart.

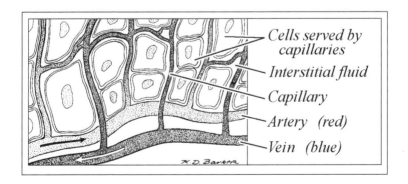

Cells served by capillaries
Interstitial fluid
Capillary
Artery (red)
Vein (blue)

Figure 26 - The systemic capillaries nourish the cells and remove their waste products.

Systemic Veins

Like arteries, veins are lined by endothelium and are made up
of three layers of tissue, but the walls of the veins are much
thinner, more supple, and less elastic than those of the
arteries. The tiny feeding vessels in the venous wall extend to
within 1/1000 of an inch of the flow surface.

The pressure is so low in veins that they don't need thick,
muscular walls. This low pressure may be the reason why
veins don't develop atherosclerosis. Arteries don't have
valves, but arm and leg veins have many valves which
prevent the blood from flowing backward when we sit, stand,
breathe out, cough, or strain.

The capillaries merge to form tiny veins that progressively
join to form fewer but larger veins until there are but two, the
inferior vena cava, which drains all the blue blood from the
lower body into the bottom of the right atrium of the heart,
and the *superior vena cava*, which drains all the blue blood
from the upper body into the top of the right atrium. From
there the right ventricle pumps the blue blood to the lungs
where it receives oxygen and turns red.

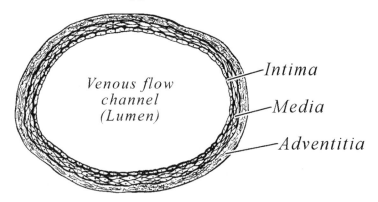

Figure 27 - Cross Section of a Systemic Vein.

Veins of the Body

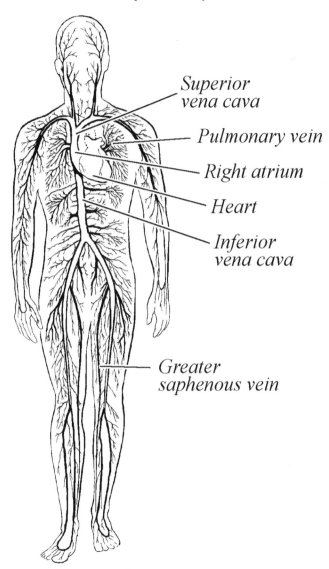

Superior vena cava

Pulmonary vein

Right atrium

Heart

Inferior vena cava

Greater saphenous vein

Figure 28 - The systemic veins return the blue blood from the tissues of the body to the right side of the heart and the pulmonary veins return the red blood from the lungs to the left side of the heart.

The force that causes the blue blood to flow back from the tissues to the right side of the heart arises from four sources:

1. The force from behind, the small residual energy remaining from the heartbeat.

2. The force of gravity in the erect position on the blood returning from the head and neck.

3. The suction force created by increasing the dimensions of the chest during inspiration.

4. The pumping force developed in the veins by the intermittent contraction of the calf muscles during walking, running, or simply moving the ankles up and down when sitting or reclining. Contraction of these muscles squeezes the thin-walled veins running between them and propels the blood they contain toward the heart as the valves below the compression site close and those above it open. Relaxation of these muscles expands the compressed veins, closes the valves above, opens those below, and literally sucks the blood up from the lower tissues.

The Venous Pump

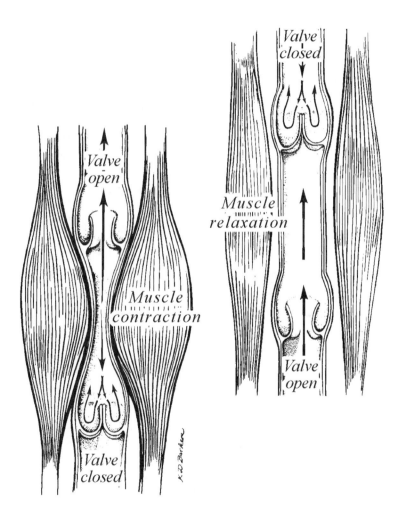

Figure 29 - Contraction of the calf muscles during walking pumps blood back to the heart against gravity.

3. Transport Medium -- The Blood

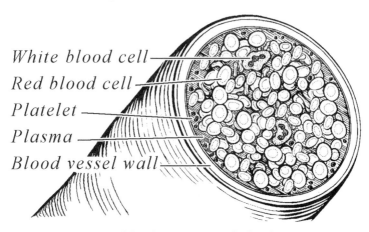

White blood cell
Red blood cell
Platelet
Plasma
Blood vessel wall

Figure 30 - Composition of Blood.

The blood is a majestic substance made up of about 40% free-floating cells and 60% fluid. Just imagine the difficulties of having to design a liquid that could carry the vast array of chemicals and huge number of cells required to nourish, regulate, and defend the trillions of cells that make up our physical bodies. Further, the blood must also be able to fill and flow easily through the 60,000 miles of blood vessels in our bodies. This distance is nearly 2-1/2 times the circumference of the earth at the equator, and is 75 times the length of the Alaska Pipeline. *And yet the average person has only about six quarts of blood with which to fill this system.* Incredible . . . but true!

The blood has huge numbers of red cells that carry oxygen to the tissues; lesser numbers of white cells (granulocytes, lymphocytes, and monocytes) that combat infection; and large numbers of cell particles, called platelets, that stop bleeding and promote healing. The red cells, the only cells in the body that don't have a nucleus, lose theirs a short time before they are released from the bone marrow.

The number of cells in the blood staggers the imagination. Conventionally, the "blood count" is expressed as the number of cells present in one cubic millimeter (mm^3) of blood. To put this into better perspective, consider what is contained in one teaspoon of blood.

One teaspoon of blood (5,000 mm^3) contains approximately:

25,000,000,000.............red blood cells
20,000,000.............granulocytes (white cells)
10,000,000.............lymphocytes (white cells)
2,000,000.............monocytes (white cells)
1,250,000,000.............platelets

If our bone marrow were to make too many red blood cells, our blood would become like sludge and cause our heart to fail. If the marrow formed too few, we would die because our blood would be unable to carry enough oxygen.

The blood cells are suspended in the fluid component of the blood which is called *plasma*. This remarkable liquid also contains most of the chemicals that are essential for our bodies to survive and function.

When an invasion of bacteria occurs, the bone marrow quickly releases a flood of white cells *(granulocytes)* into the blood. These defenders, attracted by chemicals released by the tissues, stream into the invasion area, such as a lung with pneumonia or the back of the neck with a boil, and attack the invaders. The white cells attempt to kill the bacteria by engulfing them, while the bacteria try to kill the white cells with toxins they produce. As the battle rages on, the area of combat becomes red, hot, swollen, and tender. Medically, this warfare between the white cells and the invaders is called *inflammation.*

The successful development of medicines to poison bacteria that invade the body started with the discovery of the sulfa drugs in the late 1930's. This development sharply tilted the balance of force against these invaders. Unfortunately, over time many bacteria have developed resistance to antibiotics that would have killed them a few years ago. Because of this, research teams are working intensively to develop new and better antibiotics.

Lymphocytes protect us from chronic infections and cancer. These cells arise in the thymus, spleen, lymph nodes, and bone marrow. Some lymphocytes defend us by making antibodies (special proteins that kill specific invading bacteria, viruses, fungi, and cancer cells) while other lymphocytes defend us by attacking these agents directly.

In the development of *AIDS* (Acquired Immune Deficiency Syndrome), the Human Immunodeficiency Virus *(HIV)* invades the nucleus of the lymphocytes and directs these cells to produce the deadly virus instead of making antibodies to fight the infection. Because of this, the lymphocyte count falls, and when it reaches a critical level, the patient develops debilitating chronic infections, and often cancer, too. Now largely defenseless, the patient can't fight back and usually dies within a year or two from the ravages of this disease, despite intense supportive care.

Enormous research effort is being directed to develop both an effective medical treatment and a vaccine against this dreaded disease. The need for a major breakthrough in this research is urgent because the worldwide AIDS epidemic continues to grow, especially in third-world countries. Fortunately, some progress is now being made, providing hope for the future.

Platelets are tiny pinched-off portions of the bulging cytoplasm of a large cell in the bone marrow called a *megakaryocyte.* These cytoplasmic fragments enter the blood stream and are called *platelets,* because they resemble little plates. Most float along in the circulation near the vessel wall, ever ready, should injury strike and pierce the wall, to stick together and set off a local clotting reaction to close the opening and stop the bleeding. In fact, if we were to stop making platelets, we would soon bleed to death, even from minor injuries. On the other hand, if we were to make too many, we would clot to death.

In any significant injury, vessels are damaged and some blood is lost into the wound. The platelets in the wound play two vital roles when this happens. First, they aggregate (stick together) to stop bleeding; and second, they release chemicals called *growth factors* to promote healing. These chemicals attract cells and tiny blood vessels into the wound where they multiply and heal the injury.

Monocytes are cells formed in the bone marrow and spleen that are essential to healing of a wound, control of infection, and recovery from injury. They engulf bacteria and matter that needs to be removed in order for healing to occur, and they also release growth factors that continue the healing process initiated by the platelets.

Some monocytes migrate into the vessel wall and others go completely through it to become tissue cells called *macrophages.* This name means "big eater." These cells devour bacteria, dead tissue, and clots. Like monocytes, macrophages are a rich source of growth factors that continue the tissue reaction until the wound has healed.

Blood Clotting
and
Embolus Formation

Clotting is one of the many life-preserving functions of our blood. Without this capability, we would bleed to death from even a small cut. In other words, clotting is a normal, vital, and highly desirable reaction of blood under appropriate circumstances. But clotting can also occur in the wrong place, at the wrong time, and for the wrong reason -- and can kill us by closing off a vital artery. This can happen, for example, when the tissue cap over the lipid core of a soft plaque in a coronary artery ruptures and allows the deadly fatty material to ooze into the blood and cause it to clot.

Normal clotting in an artery, such as that which occurs when we accidentally cut a finger, is triggered by the platelets, which are only about 1/5 the width of the red blood cells. Because they are small and light, platelets, for the most part, float along in the outer portion of the bloodstream close to the wall. The blood contains about one platelet for every 20 red blood cells.

But near the wall, the platelets outnumber the red cells and are ever ready to react to an injury. When the wall is injured, the platelets adhere to the damaged wall and become activated, a process which brings out their inherent maximal stickiness. These activated platelets stick to the injured area and to each other. When other platelets come in contact with these sticky platelets, they also become activated and stick to them. The process continues, forming an aggregate, a *platelet plug,* capable of closing a small cut in a little vessel.

But if the cut is too big to be closed by a platelet plug alone, platelets have another property that helps them get the job done. They can cause a protein in the blood called *fibrinogen* to form strings of sticky material called *fibrin* which sticks to itself, to the platelets, and to the injured wall, forming a multilayered mesh around the platelet plug that traps red blood cells to form a clot which attaches to the wall and attempts to span the opening. But if the clot is unable to close the opening, surgical care is required to stop the hemorrhage. If such help is not immediately available, the hemorrhage can often be stopped temporarily by applying direct pressure over the bleeding site, allowing time for the patient to be transported to a facility (hospital, surgicenter, or office) where this care can be given.

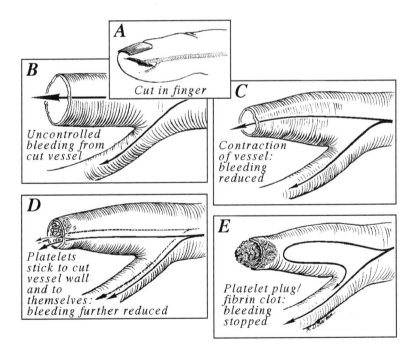

Figure 31 - Platelet plug with fibrin clot stops bleeding.

Though platelets can save our lives by stopping bleeding, they can also kill us by causing harmful clots. But platelets can only do this when they become activated and stick together. In hardened arteries, for the most part, they can become activated in one of two ways:

1. By contact with the fatty liquid that drains from the **lipid core** of a soft plaque when the tissue cap over it ruptures (see Fig. 33, p. 74).
2. By contact with the mounds of cholesterol, fatty materials, and calcium which often form the irregular, roughened flow surface of atherosclerotic arteries. Also, these surfaces frequently lose their protective covering of endothelial cells and may even develop deep ulcers. All of these changes make the diseased surfaces prone to initiate platelet aggregation and clot formation (see Fig. 34, p. 75).

Platelet aggregates or clots may cause trouble in another way. Fragments may break off and be swept by the current to a point where they become too big to go further as the flow path becomes smaller and smaller.

Such objects, called *emboli,* plug up the arterial channel at that point and block the circulation. They may be tiny and break up quickly, allowing the blood flow to resume, or they may be of such size and permanence as to cause a major stroke or loss of a limb.

Platelet emboli are uncommon in veins. Most venous emboli are clots that have detached from where they were formed in the veins of the legs and are carried by the blood to the lungs. Some of these venous emboli may be so large that they plug up the big pulmonary arteries and cause death within a few minutes from lack of circulation.

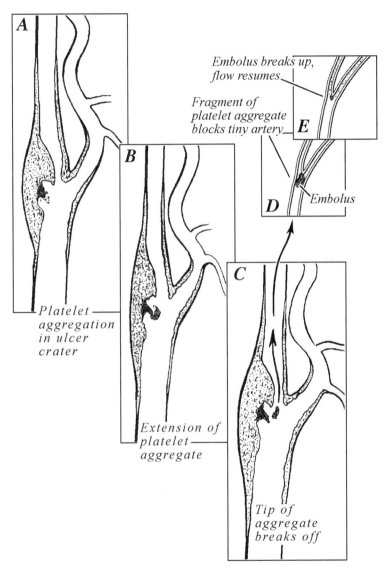

Figure 32 - Embolization of platelet fragment from ulcerated carotid plaque to small artery in the brain where it causes loss of function. If the embolus breaks up rapidly, the impairment clears quickly. Such a brief stroke-like episode is called a transient ischemic attack, abbreviated TIA.

Atherosclerosis
-- The Most Frequent Abnormality
That Affects Our Arteries --

General Considerations

In general there are *four* conditions that adversely affect our arteries. These are: injury, infection, tumor formation, and hardening of the arteries (atherosclerosis). Injury is uncommon; infections and tumors are rare. But atherosclerosis is the most frequent cause of disability and death in the affluent Western world.

Atherosclerosis is a metabolic disorder that causes the walls of our arteries to degenerate.

This degeneration can kill us in one of two ways:
1. More often, it narrows the arterial lumen (channel) and then causes clot formation which completes the closure, stopping the flow of blood to vital organs, such as the heart, producing a fatal heart attack.
2. Less often, the process weakens the wall so much it stretches, thins, bulges out, and eventually ruptures.

Atherosclerosis is caused by *blood chemistry abnormalities that result from* heredity; smoking; a low-fiber* diet high in saturated fats*, *trans* fatty acids*, sugar*, and calories; a sedentary lifestyle; excess weight; and undue stress. These blood abnormalities include:
1. High levels of one type of cholesterol (LDL).
2. Low levels of another type of cholesterol (HDL).
3. High levels of triglycerides (blood fats).
4. High levels of homocysteine (an amino acid -- see page 189).

* **Please see index and glossary**

High blood pressure, diabetes, gout, and low thyroid function also predispose us to develop atherosclerosis.

In about 5% of people, the cause of their abnormal cholesterol chemistry is *genetic*. This means that these people were born with the problem. Their livers can't remove LDL cholesterol from the blood. In the other 95% of people with hardened (atherosclerotic) arteries, the cause is due to *lifestyle* factors.

The terms HDL and LDL stand for high-and-low-density lipoprotein, respectively. Union with proteins makes cholesterol, a fat, soluble in the blood and tissue fluids. Because of its greater protein content, HDL cholesterol assists in the transport of LDL cholesterol and probably other fats out of the arterial wall to the liver for reprocessing and/or excretion in the bile. But this can't happen if there isn't enough HDL to do the job. For this reason HDL is often called the "good" cholesterol and LDL the "bad" cholesterol even though LDL cholesterol is essential to the life of every cell in the body. But as with all the body's chemicals, safety is a matter of dosage. The "bad" label for LDL is true only if its blood level is too high (above 100-120mg/dL).

Excess levels of LDL cholesterol and triglycerides saturate the inner part of the arterial wall and cause plaques (areas of marked disease) to form. Calcification occurs in and around some of these.

If marked calcification occurs, the plaque becomes *hard,* like bone. If little or no calcification occurs, the plaque remains soft. Many soft plaques develop a highly viscous, oily center, called the lipid (fatty) core. If the core ruptures into the lumen (flow channel), it may cause the blood to clot and block flow to the tissues. This is the most frequent cause of heart attacks.

Rupture of Lipid Core with Clotting

A
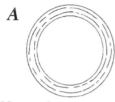
Normal coronary artery.

B
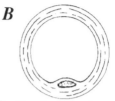
Soft plaque forming.

C
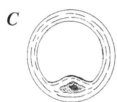
Soft plaque develops fatty liquid in central portion.

D
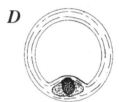
Fatty liquid core expands. Tissue on top becomes thin.

E
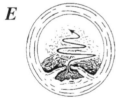
Tissue over top ruptures. Fatty liquid oozes into blood and causes it to clot.

F
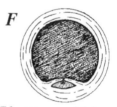
Clotting of blood continues and closes flow channel.

Figure 33 - Development of small, soft plaque with a lipid core in a coronary artery. The core enlarges and ruptures its fibrous cap, allowing the deadly, oily contents to ooze into the blood, causing it to clot. This blocks the flow channel and causes a heart attack, the most common cause of death in the U.S. If a clot-dissolving drug is given within the first hour after the artery closes, it will likely dissolve the clot, restore blood flow, and save the heart muscle.

Ulceration with Clotting

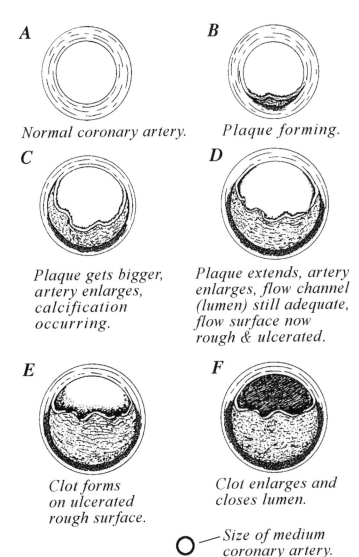

A

Normal coronary artery.

B

Plaque forming.

C

Plaque gets bigger, artery enlarges, calcification occurring.

D

Plaque extends, artery enlarges, flow channel (lumen) still adequate, flow surface now rough & ulcerated.

E

Clot forms on ulcerated rough surface.

F

Clot enlarges and closes lumen.

Size of medium coronary artery.

Figure 34 - Development of hard (calcified) plaque with flow surface roughening and ulceration in a coronary artery causes platelets to adhere, activate, and aggregate, inciting clot formation which blocks the flow channel.

Modern life in the U.S. tends to make us stressed, sedentary, and overweight. Advertisements for fast, high calorie, convenient, tasty, low-fiber, high-saturated fat, high-*trans* fatty acid, high-sugar foods are always before us. In time, our blood chemistry mirrors what we eat, what we weigh, how much we exercise, the degree of stress in our lives, and whether we smoke.

What we *should* do to preserve our arteries, the *lifelines* within us, is obvious. *We must stop smoking, eat a proper diet, exercise regularly, attain and maintain a healthful weight, and control the reactions to the stress in our lives.*

Adopting this simple prescription for heart-healthy living is the most practical way to stop the epidemic of deaths and disability that is strangling the western world. . . and increasingly, the *entire* world.

While we agonize over the high cost of medical care in the U.S., we still subsidize the farming of tobacco, and we fail to educate our children about the benefits of disease prevention. It's time for us as a *nation* to become realistic.

We must take action before the cost of our medical care becomes truly insurmountable. We can do this by decreasing the number of people who become patients and need high-tech, expensive medical care. We can make this happen if each of us will commit to the lifestyle choices that will enable us to live as healthily as possible.

There's no doubt -- our arteries are "lifelines." For when they **block off** or **burst**, we suffer severely and may die. Because of this, most of the rest of the book concentrates on the diagnosis, prevention, and surgical treatment of atherosclerosis and its complications.

Two Main Complications

For emphasis, we repeat and amplify that the two main complications of atherosclerosis (hardening of the arteries) are *blockage* of the flow channel and *aneurysm* formation. These adverse effects may be summarized as follows:

1. **Blockage of the flow channel**. The flow channel of the atherosclerotic artery may become so narrowed or even completely closed by thickening of the inner wall and formation of clots, which are triggered either by rupture of soft plaques with lipid cores or by roughness and ulceration of the flow surface, that vitally needed blood can't reach the tissues downstream. Such severe lack of blood supply causes heart attacks, strokes, high blood pressure due to decreased flow of red blood to one or both kidneys, impaired walking, and loss of limbs. These conditions are much more frequent than aneurysms and occur in higher frequency in diabetic patients.

2. **Aneurysm formation**. Here, the wall of the atherosclerotic artery, usually of the aorta in the abdomen, weakens and gives way under the incessant pounding of the arterial pressure to form a balloon-like bulge called an aneurysm. Aneurysms continue to get bigger and, usually without prior symptoms, suddenly rupture and cause fatal hemorrhage.

We will now consider how these seemingly opposite results develop.

Blockage of the Flow Channel

Atherosclerosis begins when high blood levels of LDL cholesterol, fat, and homocysteine (page 189) damage the fragile endothelial cells lining the inside of arteries. The lipids (cholesterol and fats) then move into the muscle cells in the inner part of the wall and injure them. Some die. Other muscle cells move in from the outer wall, and some of these die, too. Muscle cells around these areas of injury secrete proteinaceous materials to wall them off.

Bone-like material then forms in some of these deposits, forming what medically is called a *hard atherosclerotic plaque*. Others remain soft and some of these develop *viscous, lipid cores*. The hard plaques make the wall stiff and often brittle -- giving rise to the lay term "hardening of the arteries." The plaque process thickens the inner wall and narrows the flow channel to varying degrees.

Clots form on the inner surface of atherosclerotic arteries and block them off. The most frequent cause of such clot formation is rupture of the lipid core of a soft plaque in the inner wall of the "hardened" artery (Fig. 33, p. 74).

But clotting also occurs from platelets sticking to the rough, ulcerated flow surface of hard plaques that have lost their protective layer of endothelial cells (Fig. 34, p. 75). This clotting may be so extensive that it completely blocks the artery. The tissues that lose their blood supply die, as those of the heart in a heart attack or the brain in a stroke.

When the main artery is closed off by a clot, the only blood that's able to reach the downstream tissues gets there by going through little branches that arise *above* the blockage and join with small branches that originate *below* it.

Blockage Due to Clot

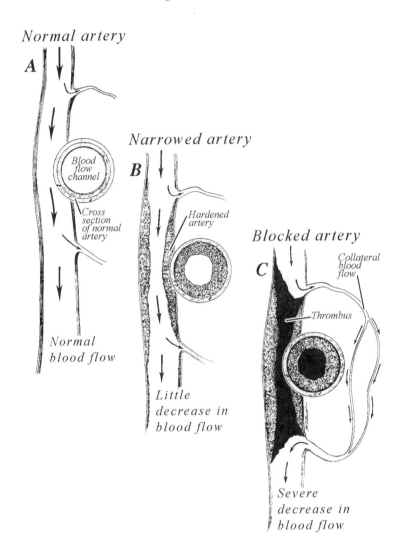

Figure 35 - Progressive Blockage of the Flow Channel. (A) Normal artery with open flow channel. (B) Development of atherosclerosis that thickens the inner wall and narrows the flow channel. (C) Complete blockage of channel by clot (thrombus) which has formed on the diseased flow surface.

Nature's Attempt to Compensate
for Blockage of the Flow Channel

If the flow channel of an artery becomes blocked *gradually,* the branches that arise immediately above and below the blockage have time to enlarge, grow toward one another, and eventually meet to establish direct connections that provide some blood flow to the tissues downstream.

The vessels that make these connections are called *collateral channels,* and the blood that flows through them is called *collateral circulation.*

Sometimes if the closure is gradual, these collateral channels may become sufficiently large that the main artery can close and the person never realizes that anything has happened (Fig. 88, p. 234). This is unusual because nature requires a long time to form channels of this size.

If complete obstruction occurs quickly, as when a soft coronary plaque with a lipid core ruptures and causes the blood to clot, a heart attack usually occurs because there isn't enough collateral circulation to supply the oxygen and nutrients necessary to keep the heart muscle alive.

Through bypass surgery, a surgeon can rapidly *create* a very large collateral vessel by placing a graft from the open artery above the obstruction to an open artery *below* it. This creates a big channel (detour) *around* the blockage and supplies blood to the impoverished tissues downstream.

The signs and symptoms of a blocked artery depend on: (1) the organ or part of the body that's affected, (2) the severity of the blockage, and (3) the degree of collateral circulation that the body has had time to develop.

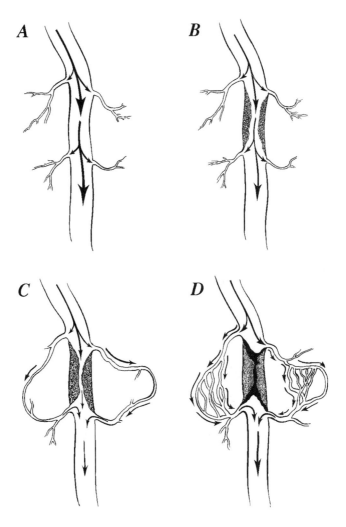

Figure 36 - Development of collateral circulation. (A) Normal artery with small branches, no collateral circulation. (B) Same artery with moderate narrowing, no collateral circulation. (C) Same artery with severe narrowing. Collateral circulation is developing. (D) Same artery, now completely closed by clot formation, with more collateral circulation bypassing the blockage. Occasionally, as shown here, substantial flow develops.

Aneurysm Formation

Even high blood pressure cannot rupture a *normal* artery because its elastic wall has plenty of strength to contain the powerful force of the heart beat.

But in some people, *atherosclerosis* weakens the arterial wall so much that the power of the pulse causes the wall to balloon out. This happens most often in the biggest artery, the aorta, more often in the abdomen than the chest, and less often in the arteries of the legs. As the dilated area (aneurysm) gets bigger, the tension on its wall increases. This increasing tension causes aneurysms to enlarge, setting up a vicious circle whereby small aneurysms get big, and big aneurysms get bigger, until they finally burst.

Though the rate of enlargement of an aneurysm of the aorta is usually gradual, with enough time, the wall **weakens** and **stretches** to the point that the arterial pressure eventually **ruptures** it. When that happens, massive hemorrhage occurs which is quickly fatal unless emergency surgery can be performed to successfully stop the blood loss.

Under the best of circumstances, the death rate for patients undergoing emergency surgery for ruptured abdominal aortic aneurysms is high . . . often above 50%. Because of this, surgery by an experienced surgeon is advised before rupture occurs if the patient's general condition is good. Under these favorable conditions, the risk of fatality is under 2%.

Differing from aneurysms of the aorta which tend to rupture, aneurysms of the leg arteries are more likely to fill with clot and close off, blocking the flow of blood.

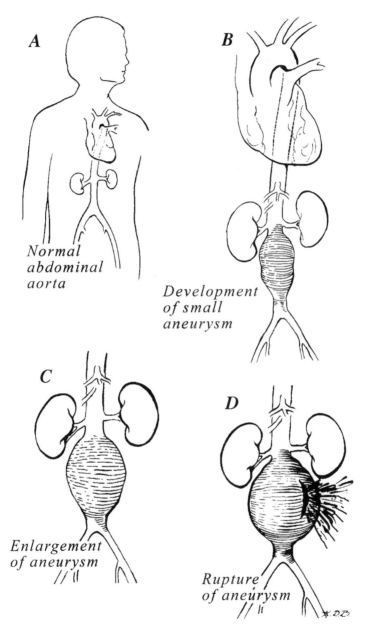

A Normal abdominal aorta

B Development of small aneurysm

C Enlargement of aneurysm

D Rupture of aneurysm

Figure 37 - Aneurysm development with progressive enlargement leading to rupture with massive hemorrhage.

Section II:
Diagnosis

Diagnosis of the Two Common
Complications of
"Hardening of the Arteries:"
1. Blockage of the Flow Channel
2. Aneurysm Formation

General Considerations 85

Diagnosis of Blocked Arteries 85-107

      Heart 88-93

      Brain 94-101

      Kidneys 102-103

      Legs 104-107

Diagnosis of Aneurysms 108-111

General Considerations

Proper treatment of a patient starts with diagnosing what is wrong. In some patients with atherosclerosis, the flow channel of critical arteries may become **blocked.** In other patients, the wall may weaken and **bulge out** (aneurysm formation). Because these events can cause death, it is important for doctors to find out (diagnose) if either or both of these threatening changes are present. This section tells how this is done.

Blocked arteries are more common than aneurysms and tend to occur where the flow channel divides, especially in the heart, neck, and legs. Such obstructed arteries may cause pain, but aneurysms seldom do until they begin to rupture. If aneurysms can be felt, they are easily diagnosed by their broad, strong pulsations. Blocked arteries on the other hand, either have weak pulses or none at all, depending on the degree of obstruction.

Diagnosis of Blocked Arteries

If narrowing of the arterial channel is marked, it severely reduces the flow of blood to the tissues and causes a threatening decrease in the supply of oxygen, water, nutrients, and other chemicals to the cells. The symptoms and changes that become evident as a result of these deficiencies depend upon which organ or body part is being deprived of its blood supply.

Blockage of the arteries of the *heart* is diagnosed by the patient's symptoms and by special studies that include:
1. Recording the electrical activity of the heart *(electrocardiogram,* abbreviated ECG) at rest and with exercise *(stress test).*

2. Determining if there is calcification in the wall of the coronary arteries by ultrafast computed tomography *(heart scan)*.

3. Performing rapid x-rays of the coronary arteries after injecting them with dye to identify blockages of their flow channels *(coronary arteriograms)*.

Blockage of the arteries going to the *brain* is diagnosed by symptoms, presence of *murmurs* and *thrills* along the course of these vessels, reflected sound wave (ultrasound) and/or arteriogram studies that outline the flow channels of the arteries going to the brain. Murmurs and thrills are caused by turbulence (chaotic, swirling flow) of the blood as it exits from a site of narrowing. In the case of a murmur, the turbulence shakes the wall sufficiently hard that the vibration can be *heard* with the aid of a stethoscope (Fig. 42, p. 97). In the case of a thrill, the turbulence shakes the tissues so hard that the vibration can be *felt* by placing a finger lightly on the skin over the artery.

Blockage of the arteries going to the *kidneys* is diagnosed by reflected sound wave studies and arteriograms. The functional significance of such obstructions can be assessed by the amount of a chemical called *renin* that the kidneys secrete into the blood. The more a kidney's blood supply is reduced, the more renin it secretes. This chemical causes the small arteries throughout the body to contract. The more renin, the tighter these little vessels constrict, and the higher the blood pressure rises.

Blockage of the arteries going to the *legs* is diagnosed by symptoms, appearance of the feet, exercise capacity, quality of pulses, presence of murmurs and thrills, blood pressure at different levels in the legs, ultrasound studies, and arteriograms.

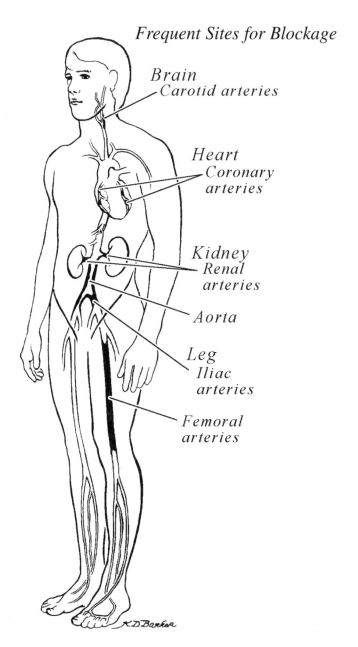

Frequent Sites for Blockage

Brain
Carotid arteries

Heart
Coronary arteries

Kidney
Renal arteries

Aorta

Leg
Iliac arteries

Femoral arteries

K.D.Barker

Figure 38 - Common locations of arterial blockages due to hardening of the arteries and clot formation.

Diagnosis of Blocked Arteries to the Heart

In years past, doctors thought that coronary heart disease was primarily a condition of men. Today, we know that this is not true. Coronary heart disease is just as common in women as it is in men, but on average it occurs about 10 years later. The reason for this delay appears to be the protective effect of estrogens (hormones secreted primarily by the ovaries) in premenopausal women.

After menopause, the lack of these hormones appears to accelerate the development of atherosclerosis. Taking a small amount of estrogen replacement daily slows this process. Estrogen replacement therapy (ERT) also decreases the severity of osteoporosis (loss of bone substance) in women after menopause. However, women taking estrogen therapy have a slightly increased incidence of cancer of the uterus and breast. Fortunately, taking a small amount of another ovarian hormone, progesterone, along with the ERT reduces the risk of uterine cancer. But because this is not so for breast cancer, ERT may not be advisable for women with a family and/or personal history of breast cancer.

Nearly 1,000,000 people died of heart and artery diseases due to atherosclerosis in the United States last year. This total exceeded the combined deaths due to cancer, infection, and accidents. Of this number, about 550,000 died as a consequence of sudden blockage of vital coronary arteries, due mainly to rupture of soft plaques with lipid cores (Fig. 33, p. 74). Many had no prior symptoms.

Sudden blockage of an atherosclerotic coronary artery by clot formation usually causes the heart muscle it supplied with blood to die because of lack of oxygen and nutrients. This event is called a "heart attack" or medically, a *myocardial infarction* or an "MI" for short.

During a heart attack, the patient often experiences severe chest pain/pressure and becomes pale, sweaty, cold, and clammy. Early in the attack, the deprived muscle, though dying, is still alive. At this point, every minute counts. If clot dissolving drugs can be given intravenously within the first hour after the pain begins, these remarkable medications can dissolve the clot that has formed over the ruptured or ulcerated plaque, restore the circulation, and save most of the threatened heart muscle.

Patients who develop severe chest pain should call for help immediately (911 in many areas) so that if they are having a heart attack, the medics can make the diagnosis quickly and begin treatment rapidly. Prompt action is often the difference between life and death.

As you can see, the diagnosis "heart attack" has become a true medical emergency because so much can be corrected by urgent treatment. Today, many patients are given clot dissolving drugs in the ambulance on the way to the hospital. In many cardiac treatment centers, patients received within the critical first hour are taken directly to the heart laboratory where cardiologists perform special studies and treatments. These will be discussed later.

Millions of people experience chest pain due to an *insufficient* supply of blood to their hearts. Most feel pain only when the heart's need for oxygen and nutrients increases, as for example, during exercise, after eating, or in the midst of an emotional upset. This pain, called **angina,** is derived from the Greek word meaning "burning sensation." Angina is most commonly felt in the pectoral region over the heart and medically is called *angina pectoris.* It may also occur in the neck, jaw, shoulders, arms, and back. In addition, some patients feel as if an elephant were standing on their chest.

Strangely, some patients with severe restriction of the coronary blood supply to their hearts experience little or no angina. Instead they *tire easily* because their hearts, which are short of oxygen and nutrients, can't pump enough blood to meet the body's needs. These patients, in fact, are in greater danger of sudden death from their hearts stopping than are those patients who, when warned by angina that the heart muscle needs more blood supply, stop their activity, place a nitroglycerine tablet under their tongue to dilate their coronary arteries, and wait for the pain to disappear.

The physician begins the evaluation of a patient who has had chest pains by asking questions about both this specific complaint and the background medical history, performing a physical examination, and ordering laboratory tests, including an electrocardiogram. Should these investigations suggest heart disease, the physician may send the patient to a heart specialist (cardiologist).

The cardiologist may order an *echocardiogram* and, for some patients, a heart scan. If the scan shows calcium in the walls of the coronary arteries, atherosclerosis (hardening) is proven. Nothing else causes this to occur.

Echocardiographic studies involve sending *sound waves* into the heart which echo back and are processed to give motion picture-like recordings of the heart's contracting ability, chamber size, wall thickness, and valve function. This study may be done at rest, during exercise, and after exercise.

The cardiologist may then decide to do a "treadmill" or "stress" test to observe the effects of progressive exercise on the patient's blood pressure, pulse rate, electrocardiogram, and symptoms. In this test, the patient walks in place on a moving surface at increasing rates and grades for specific time periods.

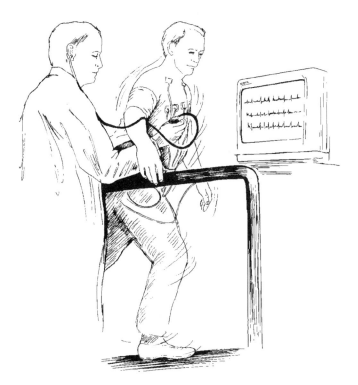

Figure 39 - Patient taking treadmill test. Physician observes patient and measures blood pressure during test.

If threatening changes occur during the test, such as a marked fall in the blood pressure; an irregular, slow, or fast pulse; major alterations in the shape of the ECG tracing; or the patient develops severe angina, weakness, or shortness of breath, the cardiologist will stop the test and note the elapsed time to when these changes began.

After termination of the test, the cardiologist observes the ECG and blood pressure and notes the time required for any stress-induced abnormalities to disappear.

Should the patient develop angina of lesser extent during the procedure that does not require stopping the test, the patient tells the cardiologist when it starts, how the pain progresses, and how long it lasts into the rest period.

If the treadmill test reveals findings suggestive of serious coronary heart disease (ECG changes indicative of a severe lack of blood supply to the heart and/or the early occurrence of marked angina), the cardiologist will probably next perform *coronary arteriograms* -- high speed x-rays of the arteries of the heart performed after injecting dye into them -- to show any blockages of the flow channels that may be present. Such obstructions may be assumed to be atherosclerotic thickenings of the inner wall which are often made worse by clot on their diseased flow surfaces.

Coronary arteriograms are performed by inserting a long, slender, hollow tube *(catheter)* into the big artery at the groin and advancing it upward into the arteries of the heart. The cardiologist then injects dye through the catheter and takes motion picture x-rays of the passage of this fluid through the coronary arteries. These films reveal any obstructions in the coronaries which block the circulation of blood to the heart muscle.

After completing the studies, the cardiologist diagnoses whether the patient has coronary disease and, if so, what is the best treatment for it. This latter decision is often reached in consultation with a heart surgeon.

Operations are advised for patients who have severe angina that can't be relieved by medical treatment and/or have arteriograms which show life-threatening blockages. Some patients are best treated by cardiologists who dilate the narrowed coronary arteries with tiny balloons attached to the ends of long, slender catheters by a procedure called *balloon angioplasty*. Other patients are best treated by surgeons who make incisions, open the chest, and implant *bypass grafts* that carry blood around the blockages.

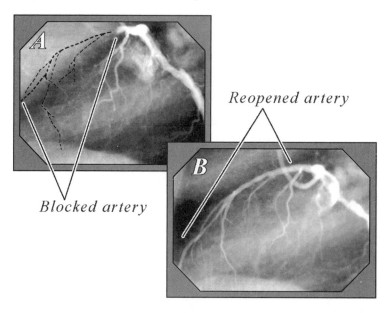

Figure 40 - Coronary angiograms showing (A) acute blockage of upper portion of anterior descending branch of left coronary artery and (B) blood flow restored in this artery by emergency balloon angioplasty.

Diagnosis of Blocked Arteries to the Brain

Two pairs of arteries supply the brain, the *common carotids* and the *vertebrals*. The common carotids are about 3/8 inch in diameter and run upward, one on each side in the front part of the neck to carry blood to the brain and head. Each artery divides into two vessels at the level of the angle of the jaw. One vessel is named the *internal carotid artery* because it goes inside the skull to supply the front and middle parts of the brain on its side. The other vessel is called the *external carotid artery* because it runs outside the skull to supply the face, mouth, ear, and scalp on its side. The division point of the common carotid arteries and the first inch of the internal carotid arteries are the sites most frequently afflicted by atherosclerosis.

The two *vertebral arteries* are the other pair of vessels that supply the brain. These arteries are about 1/4 inch in diameter and run upward, one on each side deep in the front of the neck. They pass through an opening in the side part of the upper six backbone segments in the neck and enter the skull where they unite to form the *basilar artery* which supplies the base and the back part of both sides of the brain. These vessels are less often involved by atherosclerosis than the carotid arteries.

When the blood supply to an area of the brain is blocked, its vital cells will be damaged or killed, causing loss of function. This condition, called a "stroke" or "brain attack" is caused either by fragments *(emboli)* of clots, platelet clumps, or cholesterol debris that are carried by the blood into the brain where they block vessels and shut off the blood supply; by *clots* which form in the vessels of the brain; or by *hemorrhages* from rupture of arteries that supply the brain. When this happens, the degree of brain function that is lost depends on what part of the brain was affected, how much of it was damaged or destroyed, and the effect that this injury has on the rest of the brain.

The stroke victim may be paralyzed on one side, and, in addition, be unable to feel, speak, see, swallow, smell, comprehend, perceive, or understand conversation. These and other deficits may occur in any combination and vary in all grades of severity. The loss of function may be temporary or permanent. Generally, the worse the initial deficit, the less the chance of regaining the lost function.

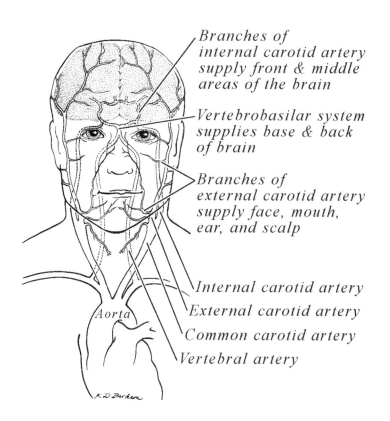

Figure 41 - Arteries of the Brain.

As with a heart attack, strokes occur when vital cells lose their blood supply and die from lack of oxygen. *Dead brain cells cannot be replaced. They are gone forever.* Hence, **prevention** of strokes, rather than treatment of their disastrous consequences, is our **primary goal.**

About 50% of all strokes occur because atherosclerosis causes the inner portion of the wall of the carotid arteries at their division point in the neck near the angle of the jaw to thicken and the surface that the blood flows over to become ragged and ulcerated.

Platelets stick to these diseased surfaces like flies to honey. These adherent platelets activate and attract other platelets which stick to them and become activated. These newly activated platelets attract still more platelets which in turn stick to them and activate, etc., etc. This aggregation cascade leads to the formation of fragile clumps of platelets that project into the blood path where small fragments can easily break off. When this happens, these particles (emboli) are carried by the blood into the brain where they plug up little arteries and shut off the blood supply to the localized areas nourished by these vessels.

Fortunately, most of these platelet fragments break up within a few seconds to a minute or two, because the lining cells of the arteries where they lodge secrete powerful chemicals which cause the platelets to lose their stickiness and separate. As this happens, the circulation returns and the stroke-like symptoms disappear quickly (see page 98). But if the fragments are large, do not break up, or do so too late, the stroke persists.

Also, when the carotid artery is severely narrowed, there is danger that the blood in the tiny opening that remains will clot and close the channel off completely. If that happens, brain cells will likely die quickly from lack of oxygen and cause a *permanent stroke.* Severe strokes usually cripple patients for long periods before they kill them.

Fortunately, these threatening atherosclerotic changes in the carotid arteries can often be diagnosed while there is still time to prevent them from causing a stroke. *Two* easy *clues* make this possible. The **first** is the presence of *murmurs* which can be heard near the angle of the jaw with a stethoscope. Murmurs are vibratory noises created by the turbulence produced when a column of blood jets out from a narrowed channel into an area of relative expansion where the flow is much slower. In general the smaller the narrowed channel becomes, the faster the blood flows through it.

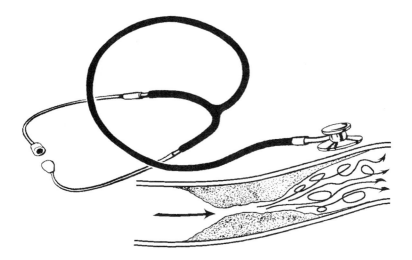

Figure 42 - A stethoscope is an instrument physicians use to hear murmurs (noises) caused by turbulent blood flow.

The **second** clue which suggests that there is atherosclerotic disease in the carotid arteries is the history of one or more brief, stroke-like episodes called *transient ischemic attacks* (TIA's). This term refers to a temporary loss of function due to a momentary interruption of circulation to a small part of the brain (Fig. 32, p. 71). The TIA may cause a brief loss of vision; sensation; the ability to speak, write, hold a glass, or walk; and many more types of deficits. TIA's get better quickly because the emboli (which cause these attacks) break up rapidly and allow the circulation to resume.

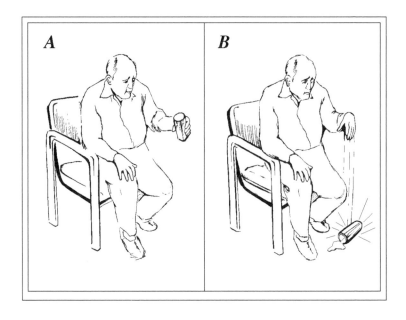

Figure 43 - This man drops the glass because a small platelet embolus to the right side of brain has caused sudden weakness of his left hand. The left hand is affected because the right side of the brain controls the left side of the body and vice versa. If the embolus breaks up quickly and allows the circulation to resume, the weakness of the left hand will disappear rapidly. In that case, the episode is called a transient ischemic attack (TIA).

Patients having TIA's are at significant risk to develop a permanent stroke in the near future. Because of this, they should contact their physicians promptly or go to the emergency room of the nearest hospital. Unless their general condition is very poor, all patients who have had a clear-cut TIA should have further studies to determine if additional treatment is required. Until recently, this meant having x-rays of the arteries supplying the brain after injecting dye into them.

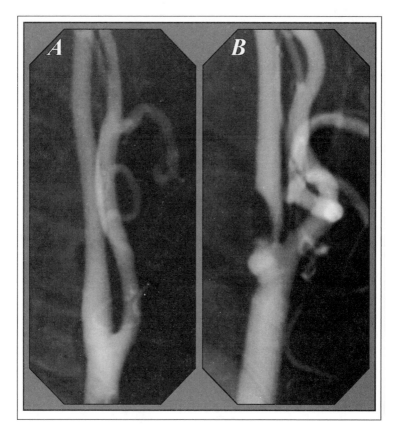

Figure 44 - (A) Normal right carotid arteriogram. (B) Abnormal right carotid arteriogram showing severe stenosis and ulceration involving the origin and first portion of the internal carotid artery.

Now, many patients who have suffered a TIA will only have ultrasound studies, usually referred to as "Doppler" or "Duplex" studies, instead of carotid arteriograms because they are also highly accurate and in addition, have no risk, are painless, and cost much less than the x-ray studies -- about $300 versus $3,000.

The patient goes to a vascular laboratory where a technician performs the ultrasound examination by passing a probe along the skin over the carotid arteries. This probe generates sound waves that are directed inward toward the underlying artery which reflects them back. These reflected waves are processed to produce an image of the flow channel.

Using another feature of this same probe, the technologist then measures the velocity of the blood as it goes through the channel. The flow becomes faster as the channel becomes smaller. This velocity measurement is an accurate indicator of the caliber (size) of the channel.

If either ultrasound or arteriogram studies show severe narrowing of the flow channel of an artery going to the brain, surgery is usually advisable, especially if the patient has had transient stroke-like symptoms. The surgeon opens the artery; removes the thick, diseased inner wall; and sutures the normal outer wall back together to restore a full flow channel that has a smooth, clot-resistant surface for the passage of blood (Fig. 79, p. 221). Most patients who undergo this operation are discharged the next day.

Carotid Ultrasound Study

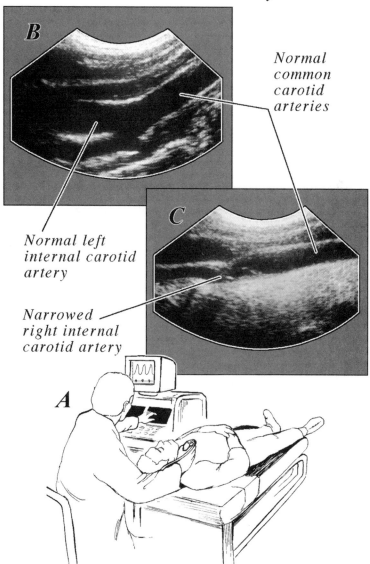

Figure 45 - (A) Patient undergoing carotid duplex ultrasound studies. (B) Normal left carotid ultrasound findings. (C) Abnormal right carotid ultrasound findings showing plaque formation with severe narrowing in first portion of the internal carotid artery.

Diagnosis of Blocked Arteries to the Kidneys

The kidneys *filter* the blood and *excrete* a yellow fluid called urine. If the kidneys are unable to do their job adequately, waste products, water, and minerals (especially potassium) build up in the blood to the degree that they may poison the body and cause death. The kidneys also secrete a hormone called *erythropoietin* which stimulates the bone marrow to produce red blood cells.

Severe blockage of the arterial blood supply to a kidney may lead to very high blood pressure (which responds poorly to drugs), and to impaired function and decreased size of the deprived kidney.

When a patient is found to have high blood pressure which cannot be controlled satisfactorily by medications, ultrasound studies and renal arteriograms may be performed to determine if there is blockage of the blood flow to one or both kidneys. When there is a severe narrowing of a kidney *(renal)* artery, the flow of blood to that kidney is decreased. This causes the kidney to secrete more of the high blood pressure chemical called *renin.* This chemical reacts with other chemicals in the blood to form a compound which causes the small arteries throughout the body to constrict. This constriction causes the blood pressure to become very high.

Severely elevated blood pressure due to increased secretion of renin or to other abnormalities can make the heart work so hard that it fails. High blood pressure also makes the patient more prone to brain hemorrhage. In addition, it may impair vision, and if due to increased renin production by one kidney, the high blood pressure can severely injure the other kidney. Though high blood pressure due to decreased blood flow to a kidney is infrequent, it must be carefully searched for in patients with severe hypertension who are resistant to medications. This is because high blood pressure due to this cause can be corrected by balloon angioplasty (dilation) or vascular surgery (removal of the thick, diseased inner wall or placement of a bypass graft to the open artery beyond the blockage). The secretion of renin by the deprived kidney decreases when its blood flow is restored.

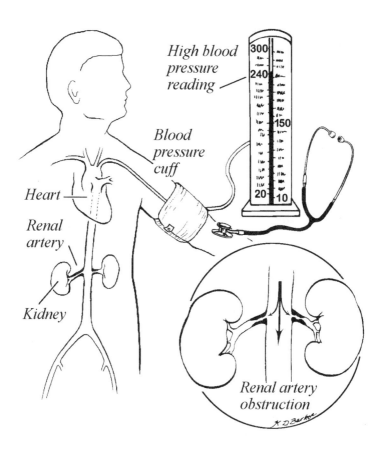

Figure 46 - Severe blockage of the blood supply to a kidney may cause very high blood pressure that responds poorly to medication.

Diagnosis of Blocked Arteries to the Legs

When circulation to the legs decreases, a sequence of characteristic symptoms begins which reflects the severity of the impairment. The first symptom is known medically as *intermittent claudication.* This means an aching pain that develops in muscles (most commonly those of the calf) that don't receive an adequate supply of red blood during exercise. The pain develops because the extra blood the muscles need to remove the lactic acid that forms during exercise can't be supplied to them by blocked, atherosclerotic arteries. When the painful muscles are rested, the volume of blood flowing through the narrowed arteries catches up with their needs, and the pain disappears, usually in a few minutes.

If the reduction of blood supply is mild, muscle pain occurs after walking several blocks rapidly or climbing several flights of stairs quickly. If the flow reduction is moderate, muscle cramping occurs after walking two to three blocks or going up a flight or two of stairs. If the reduction is severe, muscle cramping occurs after walking half a block or climbing a few stairs. Finally, if the flow reduction is critical, muscle cramping occurs after walking a few steps.

When the reduction of circulation to a leg reaches this advanced stage, another symptom appears. Severe pain now develops in the foot within an hour or two after the patient goes to bed. This agonizing symptom, called *rest pain,* occurs because the blood pressure in the foot falls when the patient lies down. The force of gravity, which helps blood reach the foot in the upright position, is lost when the patient lies flat in bed. This loss of gravitational pressure further reduces the already critically reduced flow of red blood to the sensory nerves of the foot and causes deep throbbing pain which forces the patient to try and get some relief by sitting in a chair or standing up. But the pain returns soon after the sleep-starved patient lies down again to try and get a little rest. This agonizing sequence worsens with time.

Patients with rest pain have such severe lack of circulation to the skin of their feet, especially of the toes, that it becomes pale, cold, and prone to break down and form *ulcers*. At this advanced stage, if the circulation can't be increased, *gangrene* with more tissue death, ulceration, and spreading infection is a constant threat. If this happens, the leg may have to be amputated to save the patient's life.

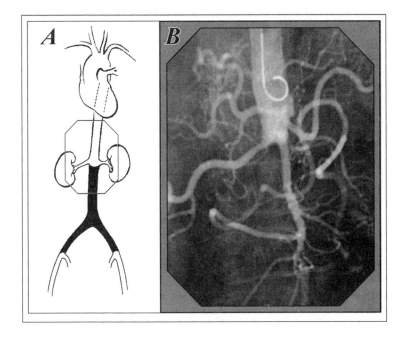

Figure 47 - (A) Drawing showing blocked aorta in abdomen. (B) Aortogram showing same thing with blockage of flow of red blood to pelvis and legs.

If physical findings suggest that arterial blockages are the reason why the patient is unable to work, can't enjoy reasonable activity, has rest pain and can't sleep, or has impending or actual *ulceration* of the toes, heel, or lower leg, a surgeon or radiologist will perform arteriograms to show which arteries are open and which are narrowed or closed. This information is essential for the surgeon to decide if it's possible to restore circulation to the limb.

Fortunately, advances in foot care and surgical techniques have greatly reduced the need for amputations. Placement of long blood vessel grafts constructed of the patient's own veins is an effective way to increase the blood supply to the lower leg, even when the graft must extend all the way from the big artery at the groin to a small vessel in the foot.

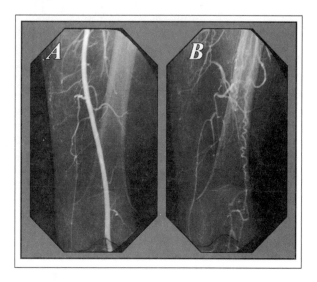

Figure 48 - Arteriograms showing (A) normal artery in thigh and (B) blocked artery in thigh that markedly reduces the supply of red blood to lower leg.

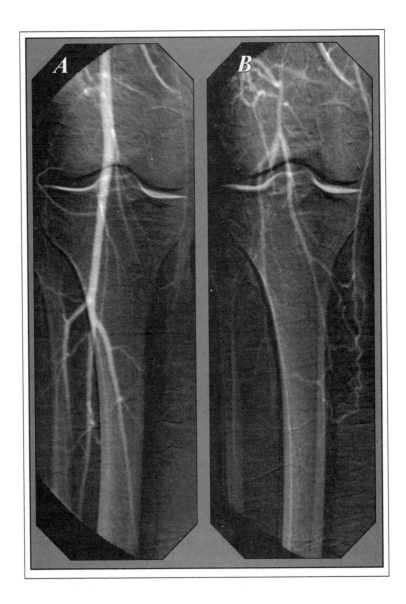

Figure 49 - Arteriograms showing (A) normal arteries at knee and (B) blocked arteries at knee that severely reduce the supply of red blood to lower leg and foot.

Diagnosis of Aneurysms

Aneurysms almost never give warning until they begin to rupture. Then the risk of surgery becomes very high. Patients with ruptured abdominal aortic aneurysms are often near death when they are brought to the hospital -- pale with low blood pressure and a painful, swollen abdomen.

Aneurysms due to atherosclerosis develop most often in the *aorta,* the body's largest artery, which emerges from the heart, arches up, slants to the left and extends backwards to descend through the posterior part of the chest (thorax) near the midline to continue into the abdomen. In the abdomen, the aorta reaches the midline at the level of the navel and divides into the right and left common iliac arteries which descend to supply the pelvis and legs below. Aneurysms develop most often in the abdominal aorta, beginning about an inch below where the arteries to the kidneys arise. Fewer aneurysms occur in the thoracic aorta and even fewer occur in the arteries of the legs.

Usually, an aneurysm of the aorta in the chest will be suggested by a "shadow" discovered on an x-ray. Further studies of the type shown on pages 110-111 are usually required to determine if the "shadow" is an aneurysm or another type of abnormality.

An unruptured aneurysm in the abdomen is seldom painful. It may be noticed incidentally by the patient who, one day, is surprised to feel a pulsating mass in the mid-part of his or her abdomen. More frequently, the pulsation will be detected by the patient's physician during a routine physical examination. Often, flecks of calcium in the wall of the aneurysm will outline its presence on an x-ray of the abdomen taken for some other reason.

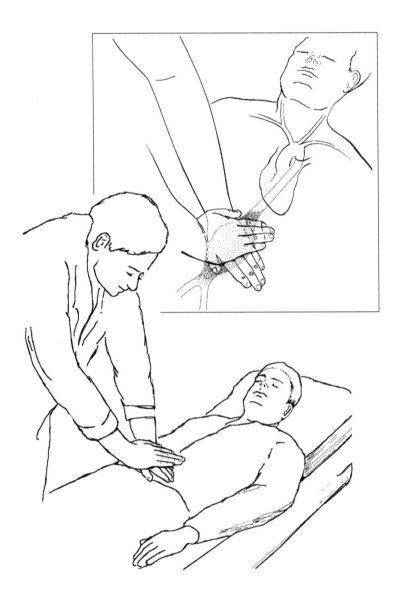

Figure 50 - Physician may diagnose an aneurysm of the abdominal aorta by feeling its prominent pulsation.

Years ago, *aortograms* were the best way to gain additional information about the aorta. No more, because CAT scans (Computed Axial Tomography) and *MRI's* (Magnetic Resonance Imaging) are technological wonders which make precise diagnosis of aneurysms easy. Ultrasound studies of the abdominal aorta are also valuable and cost much less than aortograms, CAT scans, or MRI's.

If the patient's general condition permits, the proper treatment for an aneurysm of the abdominal aorta is to replace it with an artificial artery, usually one made of

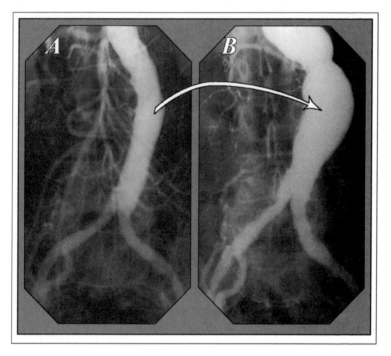

Figure 51 - (A) Aortogram showing normal-sized, elongated abdominal aorta. (B) Aortogram in this same patient six years later showing development of a bilobed aneurysm of the abdominal aorta.

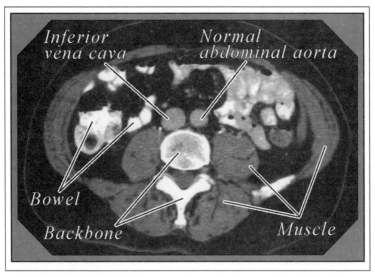

Figure 52 - CAT scan shows cross-section of abdomen revealing normal-sized abdominal aorta. (Note that the aorta is smaller than the inferior vena cava).

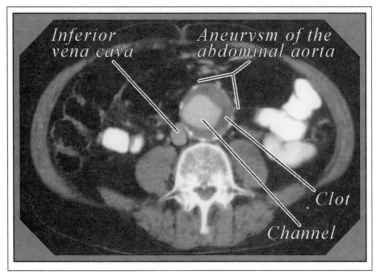

Figure 53 - CAT scan of abdomen showing large aneurysm of the abdominal aorta with considerable clot formation.

Section III:
Prevention

Prevention of Atherosclerosis and Its Complications by How We Live Our Lives

Introduction 113-115

Smoking 116-135

Nutrition 136-151

Exercise 152-179

Stress 180-181

Introduction

Some health experts estimate that up to 90% of all premature deaths due to atherosclerosis and clot formation and nearly all cases of lung cancer and emphysema could be prevented. Sound impossible? Far from it. Here's *a formula that will work* for any of us -- don't smoke and avoid inhaling other people's smoke, eat a heart-healthy diet, exercise regularly, achieve and maintain a healthful weight, and control your responses to life's daily challenges. This is good health at a bargain you can't afford to turn down.

There's little disagreement that it's how we live, day by day and hour by hour -- more than anything else -- that influences how *long* we live and how *well* we live.

And the "how well we live" is important. As we age, the quality and healthfulness of our lives becomes more important to us. We need to decide *now* how we want to live -- before it's too late to make a difference.

Having a heart attack at age 39, coronary bypass surgery at 40 and again at 48, a blocked artery in one leg at 50, an artery bypass to that leg at 51, a blocked artery in the other leg at 53, a bypass to this leg at 54, repeat operations on both legs from ages 55 through 57 to remove clots from the grafts and restore blood flow to the legs, the loss of one leg at 58, a stroke at 60, loss of the other leg at 62, carotid artery surgery at 63, and another heart attack at 65 -- with death from heart failure several months later -- is *not* the way any of us want to live or die.

Further, the monetary costs for such a person could easily exceed $350,000 -- $1 million if complications occur. Instead of such a painful and costly experience, all of us would prefer to remain *healthy* until our time to depart arrives near *age 80* or *beyond.* The primary goal of this book is to help you do just that.

But even if you already have symptoms of cardiovascular disease, don't despair, because there's an excellent chance you can turn things around by redirecting how you live your life, starting today.

Be joyful, because what you will learn in this section and the next about heart-healthy living could save your life and the lives of many of your loved ones.

Many people have been able to avoid cardiovascular surgery simply by stopping smoking and changing their eating, exercise, and relaxation habits. Others who have had to undergo surgery have avoided further surgery by making these vital lifestyle changes.

If we, as a society, do not begin to take disease prevention more seriously, medical costs will continue to rise and could bankrupt our country within 15 to 20 years.

While medical care has properly come to be accepted as a right in our society, accepting disease prevention as a binding obligation of citizenship has lagged behind. This book can help its readers correct this problem.

The challenge before us is clear. Each of us must recognize that the maintenance of our own health is a serious *personal* responsibility -- a responsibility that we owe to ourselves, our families, and our nation.

Lifestyle Risk Factors Associated with the Development of Atherosclerosis and Clot Formation

Lifestyle Risk Factors & Physiological Results	Leads to...	End Result
Smoking • Increases fibrinogen • Raises homocysteine (p.189) • Increases blood pressure • Makes platelets sticky • Restricts oxygen • Constricts small arteries	Development of hardening of the arteries and clot formation	Heart attacks Strokes
Low-fiber diet high in saturated fat, *trans* fatty acids, sugar, and calories • Raises LDL cholesterol, triglycerides, and sugar • Increases weight -- fat		Even higher blood pressure
Too little exercise • Drops HDL cholesterol • Increases fibrinogen • Makes platelets sticky • Increases weight -- fat		Heart failure
Excess weight (fat) • Raises LDL cholesterol, triglycerides, and sugar • Reduces exercise ability • Increases heart's work • Increases stress		Decreased mobility Leg amputations
Uncontrolled stress • Makes platelets sticky • Constricts small arteries • Increases blood pressure		Aneurysms and hemorrhage

Figure 54 - The lifestyle choices we make increase or decrease our risk of cardiovascular disease.

Smoking

Unfortunately, addiction to smoking occurs before its tragic physical consequences become evident. This is why smokers have so much difficulty stopping. Smokers are robbed of precious years with their loved ones, and their families and friends are robbed of precious time with them.

The *disastrous* medical *consequences* of *smoking* include:
1. The accelerated development of **atherosclerosis** ("hardening of the arteries") that leads to heart attacks, strokes, high blood pressure, decreased walking, amputations, and aneurysm formation with hemorrhage.
2. A greatly increased risk of **cancer** of the lung, larynx, mouth, esophagus, pancreas, colon, and bladder.
3. Progressive destruction of lung tissue that leads to **emphysema** and slow suffocation.

Smoking overshadows *all* other major risk factors in the development of atherosclerosis, including high blood pressure, diabetes, obesity, and blood-fat abnormalities. Even the tobacco industry now admits its product is addictive and deadly.

There's more. Mothers who smoke during pregnancy *harm* their babies. Stillbirths, premature births, low birth weight, and sudden death in the early months after birth (Sudden Infant Death Syndrome -- SIDS) are all more common when mothers smoke. And that's not all. The kidneys of some premature infants remain small and cause them to have high blood pressure as adults.

There are many more reasons why people who smoke now *should stop,* and why those who don't should *never start.*

Some Health Risks of Smoking

Shortened Life Expectancy: The risk of disease from smoking is proportional to the *number of packs* and *length of time* one has smoked. The average two-pack-a-day smoker *will die six to eight years sooner* than a nonsmoker. With these odds, why would anyone want to smoke? And there's much more.

Heart Disease: Smokers are *twice* as likely to have a heart attack and *five times* more likely to die from it than nonsmokers.

Stroke: Smoking *doubles* the risk of stroke.

Decreased Walking Ability and Limb Loss: Because smoking accelerates hardening of the arterial wall and predisposes it to clot formation, the smoker is at risk for blockage of the circulation in many areas of the body. In the legs, such blockage makes walking very difficult. The lack of blood supply may even cause gangrene of the lower legs and feet and require amputation. Limb loss is rare in people who don't smoke and don't have diabetes.

Lung Cancer: Cigarette smoking is responsible for nearly all cases of lung cancer in the U.S. Lung cancer is the leading cause of cancer deaths among both men and women. "Marlboro Men" and "Virginia Slims Women" have one thing in common . . . *they die early.*

Mouth Cancer: Smokers and snuff users have about 10 times as many oral cancers as nonsmokers. Drinking alcoholic beverages with smoking increases this risk.

Cancer of Breast: Over *half* of white American women and about a *third* of African-American women carry a gene that slows the rate of detoxification of tobacco-related carcinogens. Postmenopausal women who carry this gene and who have smoked heavily at *any* point in their lives have *four times* the risk of developing breast cancer when compared with never-smokers (JAMA, Nov 13, 1996).

Cancer of Larynx: Smoking increases the risk of developing laryngeal cancer about *five times* that of nonsmokers.

Cancer of Esophagus: Cigarette, pipe, and cigar smoking *triple* the risk of developing this cancer. Drinking alcoholic beverages also increases the risk of developing this cancer.

Cancer of Pancreas: The risk of smokers developing this cancer is *double* that of nonsmokers.

Cancer of Colon: Smoking a pack of cigarettes a day for 10 years *doubles* the risk of developing this cancer.

Cancer of Bladder: Smokers have about a *seven times* greater risk of developing this cancer than nonsmokers.

Emphysema: Smoking causes nearly all cases of this deadly disease in which the lungs lose their elasticity and become big air bags that can move little air in or out. In the advanced stages of emphysema, the patients must fight for each breath as they slowly suffocate.

Dollar Costs of Smoking

The costs of smoking in the United States are huge:

- The retail sale of cigarettes and other tobacco products is about $50 billion a year, $1 billion of which is spent by kids under 18.

- Health care costs attributable to cigarettes and other tobacco products are also about $50 billion a year.

The total annual cost of tobacco products and the consequences of their use in the United States is at least $100 billion. This figure does *not* include the cost of fires caused by smoking, or the increased cost of insurance premiums as a result of such fires. Nor does it include the cost of government subsidies to tobacco farmers. Just think of the worthwhile projects this money could be used for that would *benefit* people.

It's easy to understand why we must continue to urge those who smoke to stop, and those who don't smoke not to start. An encouraging fact is that today there are over 50 million ex-smokers in the U.S. (including 100,000 physicians).

But smoking by teenagers, especially girls -- many of whom do so in an effort to stay slim -- is increasing. An estimated 3,000 children and adolescents start smoking each day in the U.S. (about one million each year). It's not a coincidence that the tobacco industry has targeted this vulnerable group. Ninety percent of today's adult smokers started smoking *before* they reached the age of 20. Big tobacco's strategy is clear . . . *addict them early.*

How Smoking Damages
the
Cardiovascular System

Cigarette smoking increases the heart's workload and, at the same time, prevents the heart from getting the oxygen it needs to do its work. This double "whammy" is comparable to living at 14,000 feet in the Andes Mountains and having to do twice as much work as at sea level. Not a good plan.

The nicotine and carbon monoxide in cigarette smoke attack the body simultaneously in two ways to cause major heart trouble. First, nicotine increases the workload of the heart by constricting the tiny arteries throughout the body. This raises the blood pressure which increases the work of the heart and requires it to use more oxygen.

Second, the carbon monoxide in the bloodstream combines with the hemoglobin in the red blood cells and reduces the amount of oxygen that the blood can carry to the tissue cells. This also means that less oxygen is available to the heart just when nicotine is forcing it to use more.

In addition to nicotine and carbon monoxide, there are other chemicals in cigarette smoke, including millions of free oxygen radicals (page 189) that are inhaled with each puff. All of these toxic materials damage not only the lining cells and structure of the lungs but also the delicate endothelial cells that line the inside of arteries. The development and spread of atherosclerosis ("hardening of the arteries") is accelerated by each of these factors.

Smoking also increases the tendency for clots to form within arteries by making the platelets in the blood "stickier" and the level of fibrinogen higher.

Questions And Answers
About Smoking

Q. *Are people really smoking less? It seems as if everyone around me smokes.*

A. Seventy-five percent of American adults do not smoke. Furthermore, of these 150 million people, about 50 million are ex-smokers, 95% of whom quit on their own without professional help.

Q. *Tell me more about the risks of smoking.*

A. The risk of early (and painful) death increases in direct relation to the extent of smoking.

The average long-term two-pack-a-day smoker will lose about 2,500 days of life. The value of even one day of living is beyond measure. The real price of smoking can't be calculated.

Q. *Any other reasons for quitting smoking?*

A. Yes! You'll have more energy, and you'll be able to breathe easier, too.

Your sense of taste and smell will return.

If you don't smoke, there's a good chance your children won't either.

Your breath, clothes, and home will smell better.

You'll have far fewer colds and bouts with the flu,

and those you have will be less severe.

The children in your household will have fewer colds, respiratory problems, and ear infections.

Your nonsmoking spouse will not be at increased risk for developing coronary heart disease, lung cancer, and emphysema from inhaling your cigarette smoke. A real valentine.

Your home will be less likely to catch fire, and your insurance premiums should be lower.

You'll also save lots of money. If a person starts smoking two packs of cigarettes a day at 15 years of age and continues doing so for 24 years, the total cost would be about $48,000. If that money had been invested in tax-free, 6%, zero-coupon municipal bonds instead of cigarettes, the earnings of the bonds would be $96,000 during that period. The net savings would be $144,000. A nice nest egg! And even nicer if you had bought stock in Microsoft.

Q. *Tell me about nicotine, tar, and carbon monoxide.*

A. The "high" you feel when you smoke is real. It comes from the nicotine in the cigarette smoke that increases your heart rate and blood pressure. This is how nicotine addicts its victims.

A pack-a-day smoker inhales about one cup of tar each year. This terrible material contains the bulk of the cancer-causing agents ("carcinogens") that are present in cigarette smoke.

Carbon monoxide is a colorless, odorless gas which is 640 times more concentrated in cigarette smoke than what is considered safe in our nation's industrial plants. Carbon monoxide combines with hemoglobin and displaces a significant amount of oxygen in the blood, which makes it harder for the tissues to get the oxygen they need. Carbon monoxide, along with nicotine, tars, and other chemicals in cigarette smoke, accelerates the development of atherosclerosis, cancer, and emphysema.

Q. *Are smokers sick more often than nonsmokers?*

A. Yes. The National Center for Health Statistics estimates that smokers spend an estimated 88 million extra days sick in bed each year than do nonsmokers.

Q. *What are the symptoms of lung cancer?*

A. They include persistent cough, blood in the sputum, lingering infection of the lungs, and pain in the chest. By the time such symptoms appear, the chance for cure of the cancer is very low.

Q. *What is the correlation between inhaling smoke and my health risk?*

A. The more you smoke, the more you inhale. Most smokers inhale even though they aren't aware of doing so. And the more you inhale, the greater your chances are of developing coronary heart disease, lung cancer, and emphysema.

Q. *How long does it take to put yourself at risk for accelerated coronary heart disease, lung cancer, and emphysema?*

A. Experts call it a "dose-related response." That means the more you smoke the more you're at risk.

Each cigarette you smoke does some harm; the day-by-day accumulation of this damage can cause disease to develop. A pack of cigarettes a day for 15 years -- one million puffs -- will put you into the high-risk zone for coronary heart disease, cancer, and emphysema. This is Russian roulette with a vengeance. It makes no sense.

Q. *Are filter cigarettes, low-tar/low-nicotine cigarettes, pipes, or cigars safer?*

A. It was once believed that filter cigarettes were safer: after all, they were designed to help filter out some of the tar and the other chemicals in tobacco smoke. It is now known, however, that filters tend to concentrate the carbon monoxide in smoke, making these cigarettes even more dangerous than those they were meant to replace.

Studies show, too, that people who switch to low-tar/low-nicotine cigarettes often inhale more deeply and smoke more in order to compensate for the reduced nicotine.

Cigarette smokers who switch to a pipe or cigars are very likely to inhale. This keeps them at risk for the same diseases that cigarettes cause. The deadly smoke is the same.

Q. *Is the damage done by smoking reversible?*

A. Yes, to some degree. If a disease process due to smoking has not already begun, and the individual stops smoking for the next 10 years, his or her life expectancy after that period will be significantly improved. But there is less certainty about the extent of protection from lung cancer.

Also, those who quit smoking after having coronary bypass or other vascular surgery fare much better than those who don't quit.

Some harmful effects of smoking will begin to disappear soon after you stop. In weeks to months your senses of taste and smell will return, and your cough will go away. You'll feel less winded. Your circulation will improve. Your blood pressure will drop, and your heart won't have to work as hard.

Remember, you can quit for good; over 50 million other Americans have.

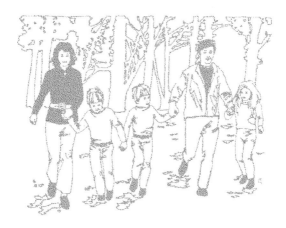

How To Quit

Ninety-five percent of those who have quit smoking have done so without the aid of an organized smoking cessation program, according to the U.S. Department of Health and Human Services. An encouraging note.

The following suggestions for "kicking the habit" have been compiled from many sources and may be what you, your spouse, or your friend need to become an ex-smoker.

Before You Quit

✔ Write down all the personal reasons you have for wanting to quit smoking (such as your health, doctor's advice, cough, smell of smoke in clothes, and cost). Read this list aloud each night before going to sleep, and read it aloud again each morning before you do anything else.

✔ Think only of the benefits of quitting. (Don't let yourself think about how difficult it might be and how many unsuccessful attempts you've made in the past.) Get excited about becoming an ex-smoker!

✔ Set a "Quit Day" sometime in the near future. (Your child's birthday, the first day of spring, or an anniversary are possibilities.) Consider your "Quit Day" sacred once you have set it, and don't let anything or anyone change it.

✔ Incorporate other positive lifestyle changes into your life. (Start by having a good breakfast each morning, taking a 30-minute brisk walk every day, eating more fruits and vegetables, and going to bed on time.)

✔ Find a friend who wants to quit smoking with you. Talk it over and plan how you'll support each other after you've both quit.

✔ Consider switching to a brand of cigarettes you dislike. Or, try switching to a brand that's very low in tar and nicotine a few weeks before you quit. This can help decrease your addiction to nicotine -- *if* you don't smoke more cigarettes or inhale more deeply to increase the "kick."

✔ Stop buying cigarettes by the carton. Wait until one pack is empty before you buy another pack. Walk to where you buy them -- don't drive.

✔ Make yourself aware of each cigarette by smoking with the opposite hand and putting your cigarettes in an unfamiliar pocket to break the automatic reach.

✔ Reach for a glass of sparkling water or spicy vegetable juice for a "pick-me-up," instead of a cigarette.

✔ Don't empty your ashtrays. The rancid smell of burnt-out cigarettes and their repulsive sight will soon disgust you and strengthen your determination to stop smoking.

✔ Don't think of quitting smoking "forever." Take it the way recovering alcoholics do -- "one day at a time."

✔ Allow yourself to smoke only in one place and don't do anything else while you do. Don't eat, drink, socialize, read, or watch TV at the same time.

✔ Open your package of cigarettes and throw one cigarette away. When you buy another pack, open it and throw two away. The key is to keep the time between packs the same while you progressively adjust to longer and longer times between "smokes." The next pack, throw three away . . . and so on. You'll have increasingly longer periods of not smoking until you just stop completely by the 19th pack or sooner.

✔ Do things that require using your hands such as needlework, craft work, crossword puzzles, or even building an addition to your home.

✔ Reorganize your life to avoid situations that "call" for a cigarette. (Go for a walk after dinner instead of watching TV. Get up earlier to avoid morning hassles. If you drink coffee, stop. Switch to tea to break the coffee-cigarette habit. Keep sugarless gum handy in your car.)

✔ Ask your doctor about nicotine replacement medications -- nicotine gum, patches, and nasal spray. These diminish the short-term symptoms that may occur when you stop smoking. You can get the gum and patch medications without a prescription.

Once You Quit

✔ Keep sugarless gum and low-calorie, crunchy foods handy such as carrots, pickles, cloves, fresh ginger, apples, and celery.

✔ A few times a day during the first week after you quit take 10 deep breaths and hold the last one while you light a match and pretend it's a cigarette. Then blow it out, and crush the "dirty thing" in your ashtray which is full of snuffed-out, foul-smelling butts.

✔ Practice relaxation techniques to reduce tension and overcome the urge to smoke. For starters, try relaxing in a comfortable chair, breathing deeply, and thinking pleasant thoughts.

✔ If you feel a really threatening urge to smoke coming on, tell yourself, "I won't give in, not now, not ever!" If the desire keeps mounting, take a relaxing hot shower and finish with a cold rinse. Tell yourself, "I can do it. I'll never go back." Then drink a glass of cold water and you'll be okay again . . . back in charge of your life.

✔ Never allow yourself to think: "Just this one time, it's okay to have a cigarette." Abstinence is the key.

✔ Avoid social situations where smoking is allowed. Instead, go to exercise facilities because they don't allow smoking, and the activities there are good for you. A hard combination to beat.

✔ When you feel tense and frustrated and want a cigarette, go for a brisk walk and before long you'll be back in charge.

✔ After a week or so when you feel in control, throw away all your remaining cigarettes, matches, ashtrays, and lighters. (Don't store them; you'll *never* need them again. Think positive. Don't waver. Remember, it's your life you're saving!)

✔ On the day you quit, make plans to keep busy. Go to a movie, take a hike, go bike riding, go to dinner . . . nonsmoking section.

✔ Buy yourself something you've always wanted, or do something special to celebrate your "Quit Day."

✔ Go to the dentist and have your teeth cleaned of cigarette stains.

✔ Drink lots of water -- at least eight glasses a day. (Try sparkling or bottled water with lemon if you don't like tap water.)

✔ Avoid alcohol, coffee, and other beverages you once associated with cigarette smoking.

✔ As soon as you finish a meal, brush your teeth. It will help break the habit of reaching for a cigarette.

✔ If you must be where you'll be tempted to smoke, associate with the nonsmokers who are there.

✔ Pay special attention to your appearance.

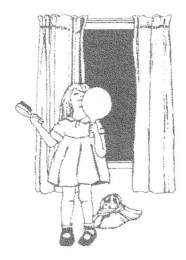

✔ Clean your clothes, sheets, blankets, pillows, draperies, and rugs to rid them of that musty, rancid smell of stale cigarette smoke.

✔ Whenever a new reason for stopping smoking flashes through your mind, write it down on your list of reasons why you'll never smoke again. Keep this expanding list on your bathroom mirror or refrigerator door.

✔ Smokers who have quit "relapse" most often during times of boredom, frustration, anger, tension, loneliness, and worry. Have a battle plan to help you through these difficult times, such as exercising, reading, calling a friend, or saying a favorite prayer.

What To Expect After You Quit

The First 12 to 72 Hours After You Quit:

You will find that these early hours are the hardest and most critical times of your battle to free yourself from the addictive grip of nicotine. If you don't stop smoking and go through this early, painful period, you'll never win your freedom. Just start and tell yourself, "I'll be okay in a few days."

During those early days you may experience shortness of breath, chest tightness, fatigue, insomnia, visual disturbances, sweating, nervousness, headaches, stomach pain, bowel upset, irritability, and an inability to concentrate.

It's important to understand that the unpleasant after-effects of quitting smoking are *temporary*. They are a result of your body adjusting to the absence of nicotine, a truly addictive drug. Maintaining a positive attitude, eating regularly, drinking plenty of water, getting extra exercise, and breathing in lots of fresh air will help you get through these difficult early days.

The First Month After You Quit:

After these first few days, you'll begin to notice some remarkable changes in your body. Your sense of taste and smell will gradually return over several weeks, and if you have a smoker's cough, it will start to slowly disappear. Your head will feel clearer -- no more headaches or dizzy spells from cigarettes. You'll be able to breathe easier, and you'll have more energy. You'll wonder why you ever started smoking, and why you didn't stop sooner.

The Second and Third Months After You Quit:

Now, the worst is definitely behind you, but unexpectedly you may experience moments of intense desire for a smoke. The aroma of fresh cigarette smoke may continue to "smell good" for several months. Don't panic. You'll be okay. These feelings will disappear with more time.

Be forewarned. When you first quit smoking, you may enjoy considerable praise and support from your friends and family. But over time, their support will decrease even though you may still be struggling, one day at a time. Be ready for this possibility and hang in there.

The Fourth Month to the Fourth Year After You Quit:

After having apparently "won" the battle, many fail here by falling into the old "one can't hurt" trap. Unfortunately, one cigarette can lead to another and in no time you could be "hooked" again. Don't give in. Ask yourself if the brief "high" provided by that one cigarette could really be worth going through all the unpleasantness and real agony of having to quit all over again. But if you should fall, don't despair. Get up and go 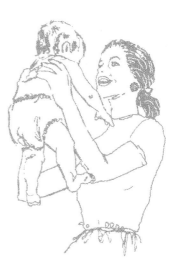 on more determined than ever to win this battle for your life. Six to eight more years of happy living with your family and friends are surely worth whatever effort it takes to permanently free yourself from this horrible addiction.

But if you *do* succumb and have a cigarette, know that the nicotine you absorb from that *one* experience is not enough to get you "hooked" again. Don't lose control. Use the "fall" as a learning experience that will prepare you to overcome future temptations.

Some would-be ex-smokers fail because they light up in reaction to every type of crisis or undue stress that develops either at work or at home. They believe that a cigarette will aid and comfort them.   The truth is, it won't. If you've recently quit smoking, decide now what you'll do instead of reaching for a cigarette when the going gets tough.

Note: Among ex-smokers who haven't smoked for five to nine years, one out of five still report an occasional craving for tobacco. It's addictive stuff, but you can beat it . . . 50 million other Americans have. They are living proof that you, too, can win your freedom.

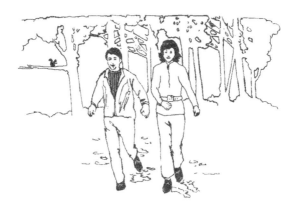

How to *Avoid* Gaining Weight When You Quit Smoking

Studies have shown that only one-third of people who quit smoking gain weight and that this group on average gains less than 10 lbs. If you have recently stopped smoking, the following suggestions will help you control your weight.

- Weigh yourself several times a week.

- Get at least 30 minutes of brisk exercise every day to reduce stress, build muscles, and burn calories.

- Read the nutrition section which begins on the next page and please follow its recommendations.

As part of a successful plan to stop smoking, some people find that "indulging" themselves a bit with an occasional special meal or tasty dessert during the first few months after quitting smoking helps them say "No" to the voice that says "Have just one, it won't hurt." They find that they can lose the few added pounds *later* when they are safely on their way to becoming a *permanent ex-smoker.*

Should you need additional help in your effort to stop smoking, please contact:

- The Hope Heart Institute: (206) 320-2001.
- The American Heart Association: (your local listing).
- The American Cancer Society: (your local listing).
- The American Lung Association: (your local listing).

Nutrition*

There are three basic types of foods: **carbohydrates**, **fats** and **proteins**. Carbohydrates and proteins are calorie poor (four calories/gram) as compared to fat (nine calories/gram).

The Standard American Diet ("S.A.D.") causes many to die prematurely. This diet has too many calories; too much saturated fat, *trans* fatty acids, and sugar**; and too many low-fiber complex carbohydrates (white bread, mashed potatoes, french fries, and white rice).

Far more important than the cholesterol we eat is the amount of saturated fats and *trans* fatty acids we consume because the *liver converts these products into LDL cholesterol.* This is the main source of LDL cholesterol.

We can limit the saturated fat and trans fatty acids in our diet by eating *little* fatty meat, poultry skin, whole milk, cream, butter, regular cheeses, rich desserts, ice cream, hard margarines, and other hydrogenated or partially hydrogenated products such as many types of crackers, cookies, cakes, candies, doughnuts, and pastries.

For most people we advise an appetizing diet, which we call the **Better Life (50-30-20) Diet©**, that gets about 50% of its calories from carbohydrates (mainly high-fiber types), 30% from fat (mainly "protective" or "good" types), and 20% from proteins that have little association with saturated fat.

---

* **See glossary for discussion of fiber, carbohydrates, fats, and proteins.**

** **The average American eats 150 lbs of sugar/year, yielding 760 calories/day or 38% of the calories in a 2,000 calorie diet. Sugar contains no fiber, minerals, phytochemicals, or vitamins -- only calories. Pop and juice drinks are full of sugar -- 10 teaspoons in a typical popular cola.**

Few carbohydrate calories should come from low-fiber sources and fewer still from sugar. Most carbohydrate calories should come from high-fiber sources (fresh fruits; fresh vegetables; legumes -- peas, beans, and lentils; whole-grain breads, cereals, and pastas; and whole grains, such as brown rice).

Most fat calories should come from monounsaturated oils (olive, canola, nut, and seed) and polyunsaturated oils (fish and vegetables -- as soybeans and corn) with not over 10% of total calories coming from saturated fats or *trans* fatty acids.

Protein calories should come from fish, skinless poultry, eggs, legumes, nuts, seeds, low-fat dairy products, and lean meat.

This high-fiber, markedly restricted sugar, low-bad-fat diet not only protects our arteries from hardening and clots, it prevents the frequent *surges in blood sugar* that tend, over time, to *cause diabetes.* These surges do this by slowly exhausting the pancreas' ability to make insulin and by decreasing the body's sensitivity to the insulin that is made.

The **Better Life (50-30-20) Diet**© is built around tasty meals of fruits; vegetables; legumes; whole-grain pastas, breads, and cereals; whole grains, such as brown rice; fish; skinless poultry; one or two eggs a day; plenty of low-fat dairy products; a small amount of lean red meat; little butter or other saturated fats; little margarine or other *trans* fatty acid products; **and very little sugar.** This high-fiber, balanced diet is appetizing and satisfying. It will help keep your heart healthy and your weight right.

The **Better Life Diet**© is for people whose livers can remove LDL cholesterol from their blood. For the 5% who lack this ability, we recommend the Pritikin or Ornish diets that limit the calories from all types of fat to 10% or less of the total.

Foods High in Saturated Fats
and
Foods High in *Trans* Fatty Acids

Restrict calories from this source to not more than 10% of total calories consumed per day.

Saturated Fats
1. Fatty (marbled) red meats and poultry skin.
2. Canned meats.
3. Processed meats such as bacon, luncheon meats, and sausage.
4. Lard and foods made with lard.
5. Butter and foods made with butter.
6. Coconut and palm kernel oils, and foods made with these highly saturated tropical oils.
7. Cream (sour/table/whipped), and foods made with cream, including rich ice creams.
8. Cheeses.
9. Whole milk, 2% milk, and foods made with them.

Trans Fatty Acids
1. Margarine* and foods made with margarine.
2. Foods made with any hydrogenated oil.

* **This spread and cooking material is largely made from soybean oil, a polyunsaturated vegetable product, that has been hydrogenated to make it solid at room temperature. But there is a downside. Hydrogenation adds hydrogen and produces trans fatty acids that are as dangerous as saturated fats because the liver converts both of them into LDL cholesterol. This becomes bad if the concentration of LDL cholesterol rises above 120 mg/dL (dL = 1/10 of a liter).**

Standard American Diet

too much...

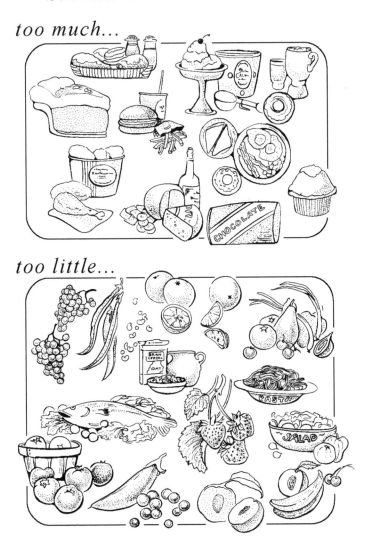

too little...

Figure 55 - The Standard American Diet has too many calories and too much of the wrong foods (low-fiber carbohydrates, saturated fats, trans fatty acids, and sugar), and not enough of the right foods (high-fiber carbohydrates, fish, skinless poultry, legumes, nonfat milk, and monounsaturated and polyunsaturated fats).

Nonfat milk is good for you. Whole milk contains too much saturated fat and so does 2% reduced fat milk. A cup of whole milk (8 ounces) has 150 calories and 5 grams of saturated fat; a cup of 2% milk has 120 calories and 3 grams of saturated fat; a cup of 1% milk has 100 calories and 1.5 grams of saturated fat; and a cup of nonfat milk has 80 calories and no fat. People who are lactose-intolerant can usually handle four ounces of milk at a meal. They can also eat live-cultured yogurt because it contains bacteria that digest the lactose.

The Goals of the Better Life Diet©

Simply put, to reduce your risk of heart disease, many cancers, and adult-onset diabetes, we advise the following dietary goals:

1. **Don't eat more** than you need to maintain a healthful weight (the weight at which you both feel and look your best -- neither skinny as a rail nor bulging out).
2. **Restrict** low-fiber carbohydrates such as white bread, mashed potatoes, french fries (which are also full of fat), and white rice.
3. **Severely restrict** saturated fats and *trans* fatty acids.
4. **Drastically restrict** sugar.
5. **Eat plenty** of high-fiber carbohydrates such as fresh fruits -- an apple a day is hard to beat; fresh vegetables; legumes; whole-grain pastas, breads, and cereals; and whole grains, such as brown rice.
6. **Choose** the protective monounsaturated (olive, canola, nut and seed) and polyunsaturated (fish and vegetable) oils within the 30% calorie limit for fats.
7. **Eat plenty** of fish and skinless poultry, but only a small amount of lean red meat.
8. **Use** nonfat or low-fat dairy products.

Who doesn't look forward to sitting down with family and friends to enjoy a great meal? No one. We all anticipate these happy occasions. It's part of our social nature. Though eating is pleasurable and necessary for life, we must be in control of what we eat if we are to live a long and healthy life. The **Better Life Diet©** is designed to do this. It deals in broad priniciples rather than emphasizing detailed calorie counting.

We can learn much about the importance of diet and habits from studies of select population groups. For example:

> Seventh-Day Adventists who restrict or avoid meat, tobacco, and alcohol have much less heart disease, lung cancer, emphysema, and liver disease than the general population.

> Deaths from breast and colon cancer are uncommon in countries where the diet is low in animal fat.

> Japanese emigrants to the U.S. who adopt our low-fiber, high-saturated fat, high-*trans* fatty acid, high-sugar Western diet are at higher risk to develop coronary heart disease, diabetes, and breast and colon cancer than are the Japanese in Japan who eat their traditional high-fiber, low-saturated fat, low-sugar native diet.

Compared with people of normal weight, obese people have a higher incidence of heart disease, diabetes, cancer (prostate and breast), and gall bladder disease.

Proteins - 20%
- Fish
- Skinless poultry
- Eggs
- Legumes
- Nuts and seeds
- Low-fat dairy
- Lean Meat

`4 cal/gm`

Fats - 30%

`9 cal/gm`

- 2/3 or more from mono and polyunsaturated fats (see page 137)
- 1/3 or less from saturated fats and *trans* fatty acids (see page 138)

High-Fiber Carbohydrates - 50%

`4 cal/gm`

- Fresh Fruits
- Fresh Vegetables
- Legumes - - Peas, Beans, and Lentils
- Whole-Grain Breads, Cereals, and Pastas
- Whole Grains such as Brown Rice

*Figure 56 - Building Block Diagram of the **Better Life Diet**©
reflects a calorie origin of 50% from carbohydrates (mainly high-
fiber types), 30% from fats (mainly mono and polyunsaturated
types), and 20% from proteins that have little association with
saturated fats. Also see page 145.*

The shape of the **Better Life Diet**© Building Block Diagram accurately reflects the origin of calories from carbohydrates (50% - 4 cal/gm), fats (30% - 9 cal/gm), and proteins (20% - 4 cal/gm). For a 2,000 calorie daily intake, this means 250 grams of carbohydrates, 67 grams of fat, and 100 grams of protein.

The **Better Life Diet**© emphasizes high-fiber carbohydrates; unsaturated fats; and proteins from fish, skinless poultry, eggs, legumes, nuts, seeds, low-fat dairy products, and lean meat. This diet calls for a restriction in low-fiber carbohydrates, a severe restriction in saturated fats and *trans* fatty acids, and a drastic reduction in sugar.

This diet assures an adequate supply of fiber, minerals, phytochemicals, and vitamins. Also, the **Better Life Diet**© markedly reduces the sugar stimulus for insulin secretion which protects against the development of adult-onset diabetes, obesity, and hardening of the arteries.

Comparable Servings for the Different Types of Foods

Pastas, Breads & Cereals
- 1/2 cup cooked pasta
- 1 slice bread
- 1 medium muffin
- 1/2 bagel or English muffin
- 4 small crackers
- 1 tortilla
- 1/2 cup cooked cereal
- 1/2 cup cooked rice

Fruits
- 1 whole medium fruit like an apple, pear, or peach (about 1 cup)
- 1/4 cup dried fruit
- 1/2 cup canned fruit
- 1/2 to 3/4 cup fruit juice

Vegetables & Legumes
- 1/2 cup cooked vegetables or legumes
- 1/2 cup raw chopped vegetables
- 1 cup raw leafy vegetables
- 1/2 to 3/4 cup vegetable juice

Meat & Meat Alternatives
- 2 to 3 oz. (size of a deck of cards) cooked *lean* meat, skinless poultry, or fish*
- 2 eggs
- 7 oz. tofu
- 1 cup cooked legumes (dried beans or peas)
- 1/2 cup nuts or seeds

Milk & Milk Products
- 1 cup (8 oz.) whole milk or whole milk yogurt**
- 2 slices cheddar cheese, 1/8" thick (1 oz.)**
- 2 cups creamed cottage cheese**

* **Most of the fat in fish, especially salmon, tuna and trout, is protective of our arteries. Because of this, fish should be eaten in preference to lean red meat or pork.**

** **Should be avoided because they are high-calorie/high-saturated fat. Use low-fat/nonfat varieties.**

How Many Servings Do **You** Need Each Day?

Calorie Level[1]	Children, Women, Older Adults About 1,600	Teen Girls, Active Women, Most Men About 2,200	Teen Boys, Active Men* About 2,800
Milk &Milk Products Group[2]	2 to 4	2 to 4	2 to 4
Meat & Meat Alternatives Group	2	2	3
Vegetable and Legume Group	3	4	5
Fruit Group	2	3	4
Bread and Cereal Group	6	9	11
Total Fat (grams) [3]	53	73	93

* **Girls and women of comparable size, muscle mass, and activity level need the same number of calories as teen boys and active men.**

[1] **These are the calorie levels** if you choose *nonfat, lean* foods from the five major food groups and restrict foods with lots of saturated fat, *trans* fatty acids, and sugar.

[2] **Teens, young adults, pregnant and nursing women, and women** concerned about osteoporosis prevention need at least 4 servings (or additional calcium from alternative sources)

[3] **Number of grams of fat when 30% of daily calories are from fat sources.**

People who store excess fat around their waists have a significantly higher risk of high blood pressure, diabetes, early heart disease, and certain types of cancer than people who store excess fat around their hips and thighs. Should you have an expanded waist line, it is especially important that you follow the guidelines given in this book.

The **Better Life Diet**© advises 30% of total calories* from fat but not more than 10% from saturated and *trans* fatty acid sources with the rest from unsaturated fats (oils) that protect our arteries such as those found in olives, canola seeds, other seeds, nuts, fish, and soybeans. But even though these fats are good for us, they, like all fats, are so high in calories (9/gram) that they must be taken in moderation. Also, the **Better Life Diet**© requires a **drastic**** reduction in sugar for the reasons given on pages 136-137.

  * **We advise the more restrictive Pritikin or Ornish diets (10% or less of total calories from fat) for the 5% of patients with a "gene" problem who have LDL cholesterol levels above 300, a low HDL, and a family or personal history of early heart attacks, often before age 40.**

** **Sugar (glucose) is the primary stimulus for insulin secretion by the pancreas. Insulin enables all the cells of the body to use glucose for energy. Insulin also causes glucose to be stored as glycogen, converts glucose into fat when the limited glycogen sites are filled, and acts to prevent fat from being used for energy. The up-and-down sugar-insulin relation fans the appetite; fats and proteins supress it. Eating sugar throughout the day makes the sugar-fat pathway a one-way street -- fat in, no fat out. Drastically reducing sugar in the diet lowers insulin secretion and acts to prevent obesity, diabetes, and athersclerosis.**

  By all but deleting table sugar, standard soft drinks (pop), "juice" drinks, jams, jellies, candies, cakes, pies, pastries, ice creams, and many other desserts, the average daily consumption of sugar on a 2,000 calorie diet can be easily reduced from about 190 grams (760 calories, 0.42 lb)to about 60 grams (240 calories, 0.13 lb).

21 Ways to Lower
The Saturated Fat and *Trans* Fatty Acid
Content of Your Diet

1. Use a nonstick cooking spray and a nonstick frying pan instead of adding butter or margarine for frying.

2. Remember, the word "imitation" in the case of dairy products isn't necessarily bad because it usually means that the saturated fat content is lower than it is in the standard product. (Read the labels to be sure.)

3. Select red meat with the least fat. "Prime" grade has the most fat, "choice" less, and "good" still less.

4. Trim away all visible fat on red meat before cooking or eating. You can literally save hundreds of calories by removing this store of saturated fat.

5. Remove poultry skin and attached fat (saturated) before cooking. (Most of the poultry fat lies just under the skin.)

6. Prepare foods in which the fat cooks into the liquid (stews, boiled meats, and soup stock) a day ahead of time. Then chill the food and remove the fat (mainly saturated) which rises to the top and hardens.

7. Add a few ice cubes to meat drippings to harden the fat. This will allow you to make a low-fat gravy. The fat (mainly saturated) will cling to the ice cubes.

8. Use low-fat yogurt on potatoes instead of butter or margarine.

9. Beware, a salad-bar salad can have more calories than a fatty entree. Watch the salad dressings (70 to 100 calories per tablespoon); marinated vegetables; and mayonnaise-laced pastas, meats, and cheeses.

10. Brown meats under the broiler rather than on the stovetop. No additional oil is required, and the liquified fat will drip into the pan below.

11. Reduce the amount of fat in canned meats, broths, and stews, by chilling the cans before opening them. After being chilled, it's easy to skim off the fat (mainly saturated) which has risen to the top and solidified.

12. Substitute mustard, ketchup, relish, and/or salsa for butter and margarine in sandwiches.

13. Don't eat turkey only at Thanksgiving -- eaten without the skin, it's low in fat and good throughout the year.

14. Microwave, bake, broil (on rack), poach, or stir-fry foods instead of frying.

15. Use either canola or olive oil for cooking and salads because both of these oils contain more protective monounsaturated fats than any other such agent.

16. Cook bacon and other fatty breakfast meats well, and then press them firmly between absorbent paper towels to remove as much of the remaining fat as possible before eating these foods.

17. Limit red meat to three 3-ounce servings of lean varieties a week. Eat more fish, poultry (without skin), legumes, and nonfat dairy foods.

18. Switch from whole milk or 2% milk, to 1% or nonfat milk. Whole milk will taste unbearably thick and fatty once you're used to nonfat milk. Your taste preference will change in several weeks.

19. Select the softer margarines because they have fewer *trans* fatty acids. Squeezable liquid margarines have the least and stick margarines the most. Tub margarines have an intermediate amount of these "bad" fatty acids.

20. Select hamburger that is labeled "extra lean" and cook it under the broiler to remove more fat.

21. Buy low-fat ("light," "diet," or "skim") cheeses, instead of regular cheeses.

For more dietary information we recommend the following resources:

- *Dr. Atkins New Diet Revolution* by Robert C. Atkins, MD. Available at your local bookstore.

- *Dr. Dean Ornish's Program For Reversing Heart Disease.* Available at your local bookstore. Call (800)775-7674 to be put on Dr. Ornish's mailing list for free information about his programs and research.

- *Don't Eat Your Heart Out Cookbook* by Joseph C. Piscatella. Available at your local bookstore.

- Pritikin Longevity Center
  Santa Monica, CA
  Call (800) 421-9911 for free videos and diets.

Basics for Weight Control

The body can store little protein or carbohydrate (glucose). In fact, less than a pound of glucose (as glycogen) can be stored in the entire body, 1/3 in the liver and 2/3 in the muscles. But the body is very efficient at converting extra protein* and carbohydrate (glucose) into saturated fat. Furthermore, the body has an almost limitless capacity to store fat in the cells of the adipose tissue throughout the body.

Sugar stimulates the pancreas to secrete insulin. Insulin converts the extra sugar into fat and acts to keep it there -- a one way street -- by blocking the use of fat for energy.

If low-fiber carbohydrates are restricted and sugar is drastically reduced, weight control becomes relatively easy for most people. But if these foods along with fats are consumed without restraint, obesity becomes a certainty along with a clear predisposition to diabetes and heart disease. This is so because sugar fans the appetite and *excess sugar* (beyond the limited amount that can be stored as glycogen) is *converted* into *fat.*

The **Better Life Diet**© provides a balanced intake of carbohydrates, 50% (mainly high-fiber), fats, 30% (mostly the protective unsaturated types), and proteins, 20% (with little saturated fat), to supply the energy, building materials, fiber, minerals, phytochemicals, and vitamins needed by our bodies.

The building block diagram of the **Better Life Diet**© on page 142 is a guide for developing such a balanced diet. The number of servings you require from each group depends on your caloric needs to maintain a healthy weight, page 145.

---

* **Amino acids (from protein) are converted into glucose.**

How to Lose Excess Weight

Obesity (excessive accumulation of fat) makes the heart work harder and produces biochemical changes (see page 115) that cause arteries to wear out.

Many people eat too much, don't exercise enough, and put on excessive weight (fat). Losing this fat requires special knowledge. Losing weight is a matter of eating the *right foods* in the *proper amounts* and *exercising* (see next page). Without proper exercise and an adequate protein intake, more muscle will be lost than fat. Crash diets *aren't* the answer. In the inevitable relapses that follow these diets, more fat is added than muscle. The *result* is a heavier, weaker, and fatter person who wonders what went wrong.

The answer is to add muscle and lose excess fat. This means that the overweight person must get some calories by using up part of their fat stores every day. This happens when one eats fewer calories than he or she uses.

Fats and proteins suppress the appetite while sugar increases it in a cyclic manner by stimulating insulin formation. Person eats sugar; blood sugar rises; more insulin secreted; appetite decreases for a short time; blood sugar falls; less insulin secreted; appetite increases; person eats more sugar; the cycle repeats. This is why the key to losing weight is to restrict the low-fiber carbohydrates (rapid source of glucose) and drastically reduce sugar in the diet.

The **Better Life Diet**© combined with a consistent exercise program and about a 20% decrease in calories will cause loss of 1/2-to-1 lb/wk. When the target weight is reached, the exercise program is continued and the diet is returned to a caloric intake that will maintain this desired weight.

Exercise

Aerobic ("with oxygen") exercise is rhythmic muscular activity performed at a pace that is within the capacity of the circulation to deliver needed oxygen to and remove excess carbon dioxide from the working muscles. You can continue this exercise for long periods with a stable, moderately elevated pulse rate without becoming breathless, exhausted, or drenched in sweat. This exercise is safe and good for you. It's the exercise you need to become healthy and stay that way.

On the other hand, anaerobic ("without oxygen") exercise demands more oxygen than the arterial blood can deliver to your muscles. Such exercise makes you severely short of breath, causes your pulse to race, and wears you out quickly. And unless you're a trained athlete, it's neither good nor safe for you.

To benefit your heart, exercise must be aerobic. If you can carry on a normal conversation while exercising, that exercise is aerobic for you. Aerobic exercise *doesn't* deplete you of oxygen, make you short of breath and unable to talk,or cause you to perspire heavily (unless it's very warm). On the other hand, anaerobic exercise *does* deplete you of oxygen, make you breathless and unable to speak, and cause you to perspire heavily.

The ability to talk while exercising (the talk test) is as simple way to tell whether an exercise is "aerobic" for you. If you can talk, it is; if you can't, it's anaerobic. People in poor shape fail the test while walking slowly; people in good shape pass while walking briskly; people in excellent shape pass while jogging. Regardless of the activity, adjust your pace so you can pass the "test."

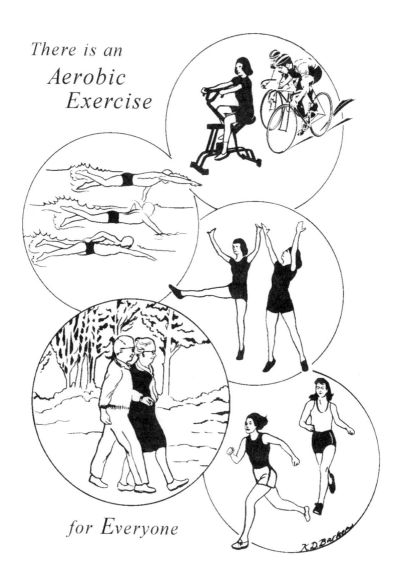

Figure 57 - Aerobic exercise is good "every day medicine."

Aerobic exercise costs little in time or money, and it greatly increases your enjoyment of life. Such exercise tones your muscles, sharpens your mind, strengthens your heart and lungs, helps your whole body use oxygen and nutrients more efficiently, assists and encourages you to maintain a healthy weight, reduces stress, alleviates depression, and improves dangerous blood chemistry.

In brief, regular aerobic exercise is the closest thing we have to an "anti-aging pill." You'll find that life's a lot more fun when you take this "pill."

Regular aerobic exercise also helps the digestive system work better; promotes sound sleep; and together with proper diet, vitamin D, calcium, magnesium, and estrogen in women (after menopause) acts to prevent or at least slow down the development of osteoporosis, a condition that absorbs bone structure and weakens the skeleton.

Severe osteoporosis weakens the long bones so much that they break easily, especially the hip, and makes the backbone so fragile that portions of it may collapse. Even without obvious fractures, osteoporosis silently shortens the spine with age and causes both men and women to lose height as they get older.

We all need aerobic exercise. Not only can it help us lose excess body fat, it strengthens our muscles, gives us a renewed sense of vigor, and helps protect us from atherosclerosis with its complications of heart attack, stroke, high blood pressure, impaired mobility, limb loss, and aneurysm formation with rupture.

Walking as briskly as possible without becoming winded is hard to beat as an exercise for many reasons. It's safe, pleasant, inexpensive, good for most everything, and able to be enjoyed nearly any time and any place. Try it! Two miles in the morning and/or evening will do wonders for you. This is a habit to form and practice for life.

Walk with your husband, wife, children, friend, or dog. If none of them are available, walk alone. This is time you owe yourself. Precious time.

If you can't walk two miles, try one. If not one, do what is comfortable for you and slowly increase the distance.

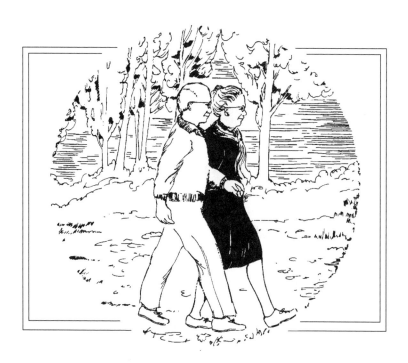

Figure 58 - Walking is an exercise that's possible for most everyone.

F.I.T.

The Basics - Think F.I.T.

The first thing to know about "regular aerobic exercise" is that unless you do it *frequently enough, intensely enough,* and *long enough,* it's not going to do you, your cardiovascular and respiratory systems, or your weight reduction program much good.

As an aid to getting in shape and staying that way, think F.I.T. for the **frequency**, **intensity**, and **time** of exercise.

Frequency

The American College of Sports Medicine recommends that people get some exercise every day of the week. We need to use our muscles consistently (like every day) to keep them and our heart and lungs in shape. There's no way around this requirement. We either use our muscles or we lose them. An easy choice.

Intensity

Most of the mystique that surrounds aerobic exercise has to do with its intensity, or "pace."

Take the "talk test" to find the aerobic pace that's right for you (page 152). Increase your pace to where you can't carry a conversation and then back off to where you can. In doing this, don't try to exercise on the "edge." Give yourself some "breathing room."

When you're in the "groove," you'll work up a moderate sweat, but you won't get breathless. If you find yourself huffing and puffing and unable to speak, slow down and find the pace that's right for you.

Time

Studies show that for reasonable fitness, we need at least 30 minutes of aerobic exercise every day of the week.

There is some controversy here. A panel of experts convened by the American College of Sports Medicine and the Centers for Disease Control (CDC) recently announced that *accumulating* 30 minutes of "moderate exercise" each day (e.g., walking, gardening, climbing several flights of stairs and/or doing housework *every* day) is enough to improve overall fitness, at least moderately.

But researchers at the Harvard School of Public Health believe that 45 minutes of daily, brisk, *continuous* exercise is preferable.

The bottom line is that even a *little* exercise is better than no exercise, and in general, *more* exercise is better than less exercise -- within reason of course.

Although 30 minutes of daily aerobic exercise can help you in terms of cardiovascular fitness, it won't burn off a lot of calories.

Serious weight watchers should plan on getting at least 45 to 60 minutes of continuous, brisk aerobic exercise everyday. *It works!*

Questions and Answers
About Exercise

Q. *What are the different types of exercise?*

A. 1. Isometric exercise (muscle contraction without motion) tones your muscles, but doesn't move your body around. This type of exercise uses few calories and doesn't improve overall cardiovascular and muscular fitness.

2. Isotonic exercise -- such as weight lifting -- builds muscle tissue and uses calories but doesn't do enough for your cardiovascular or pulmonary fitness.

3. Anaerobic exercise *(without* adequate oxygen) -- such as sprinting or fast cycling -- leads to exhaustion and breathlessness in a few minutes. This type of exercise can't be continued long enough for needed benefits to be realized. Also, anaerobic exercise is dangerous because it quickly depletes your heart of oxygen.

4. Aerobic exercise *(with* adequate oxygen . . . if your pace is right) such as walking, dancing, jogging, cycling, swimming, handball, tennis, rowing, and rope skipping are the most popular. At a proper aerobic pace, these exercises build muscle, get your heart and lungs in shape, help you attain and maintain a healthful weight, and keep you in good condition. This combination of benefits could save your life.

Q. *Should I check with my doctor before beginning an exercise program?*

A. Yes, if you:
- Haven't seen your doctor for a long time.
- Are over 35 years of age.
- Have a personal or family history of cardiovascular disease.
- Are a smoker.
- Have high blood pressure.
- Are seriously overweight.

Q. *How do I know which aerobic exercise is best for me?*

A. Considerations for choosing an aerobic exercise (or a combination of aerobic exercises) should include:
- The availability or price of equipment purchase or rental.
- Your personal health, weight, and age.
- Your level of fitness.
- Your interests.
- The weather.
- How much time you have.

Q. *How can I find time to exercise?*

A. The same way you find time every day to eat and sleep. Exercise is just as important. Make it a priority.

Q. *What are my exercise choices?*

A. There are many. The following comments about the more popular aerobic exercises are to pique your interest and get you involved.

1. Aerobics

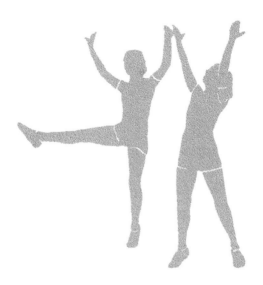

Special Advantages:
- Special fun for those who like exercising to music.
- Entire body is exercised.
- Group spirit is established in the classes.
- Necessary skill is rapidly acquired. Beginners become "pros" in a short time.
- Classes are held inside, away from the weather.
- Many styles of aerobics and different kinds of music to choose from.

Special Equipment/Facilities Needed:
- Loose-fitting clothing and comfortable shoes with cushioned soles (athletic shoes give the best support).
- Space and a qualified instructor.

Advice for Beginners:
- The best way to find a good aerobics program and instructor is by word-of-mouth referral. Talk to your friends and find out what program and which instructor they enjoy and why. If that doesn't work, check with the registered programs (as at the YWCA or YMCA) in your community and ask what they offer. Then talk to their instructors.

- Sign up for classes with a friend. You'll push each other and have a lot of fun doing so.

- Aerobics classes that are only offered twice a week don't provide enough exercise to get your cardiovascular and respiratory systems in good shape. To get more exercise, sign up for two programs, or supplement your classes with other aerobic exercises that you do on your own, such as walking or swimming.

- The typical aerobic dance program consists of a one-hour class Monday, Wednesday, and Friday for three months.

- Make sure you exercise strenuously enough in your class to work up a sweat, but don't get so carried away that your pace causes you to become breathless and drenched in sweat.

2. Cycling

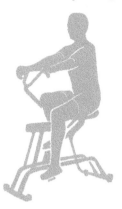

Special Advantages:
- Especially well-suited for older and overweight individuals, as well as for those with back, knee, and/or foot problems.

- Outdoor bikes can be used for transportation.

- Indoor bikes provide protection from the weather, and you can read or watch TV while exercising.

Special Equipment Needed:
- An outdoor or indoor bike. These may be purchased or rented from a cycle shop. Want ads and garage sales may be useful in finding a good second-hand bike.

- Before purchasing a bike, check consumer magazines and bicycle books, talk with friends, and, if you still need more guidance, consult a fitness professional. Then, comparison shop.

- Outdoor bikes should have at least three gears.

- Indoor bikes must have a tension control -- all other special features are optional.

Advice for Beginners:
- Work on finding a pedaling pace appropriate for your fitness level that will give you an adequate workout without causing shortness of breath. If you get to a point of breathlessness, slow down until you catch your breath. Then pick your pace up to the point you're sweating some but aren't winded.

- Have a bike specialist "fit" your bike to your body by adjusting the seat and handle bar height and position so your legs and back are comfortable.

- Outdoor cyclists should wear helmets because they provide needed protection which could prevent a devastating head injury in case of an accident.

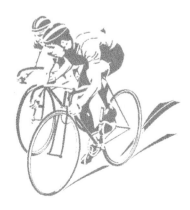

3. Swimming

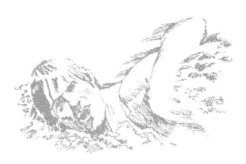

Special Advantages:
- Well-suited for everyone and especially those with back and/or joint problems which restrict or prohibit them from enjoying other popular aerobic exercises.

- The perfect aerobic exercise for those who want a good workout but hate to sweat.

- Works on all body muscles.

Special Equipment/Facilities Needed:
- Swim suit.

- Eye and ear protection, if necessary.

- A swimming pool. If you don't own one, check out the parks department pools, or the pool at the YMCA, YWCA, or local health club. Be sure the pool is large enough for nonstop lap swimming.

Advice for Beginners:
- Inquire when your local pool opens for lane swimming. Some pools are open from 5:00 A.M. to 10:00 P.M.

- Use any stroke and get in as much nonstop lane swimming as possible during your exercise time. If you start to lose your breath, switch to a lazy sidestroke. Once you've caught your breath, find your proper pace.

- If it's difficult for you to get to a pool on a regular basis, use the other suggested aerobic exercises to supplement your swimming program.

Swimming and Osteoporosis:
- Studies have shown that swimming *doesn't* help strengthen bones. If you're concerned about osteoporosis, get plenty of *weight-bearing* exercise, like walking.

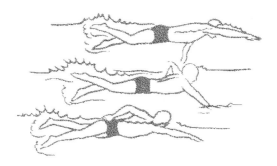

4. Walking

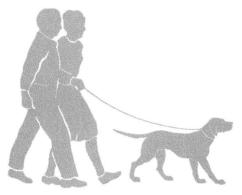

Special Advantages:

- Good way to begin an exercise program if you haven't been exercising, have special medical problems, and/or are overweight.

- Can be used to limber up sore muscles if you've "overdone it" with one of the other aerobic exercises.

- Can be used for transportation.

- Can provide the same benefits as jogging, with less risk of injury.

- No expertise needed; you've been doing it since you were one year-old.

Special Equipment Needed:

- Comfortable shoes with cushioned soles.

Advice For Beginners:

- If you're out of shape, begin slowly and first increase the distance and then your pace, but do this in a careful, progressive manner. If you become breathless, you're going too fast . . . slow down! When you've caught your breath, continue at a pace that enables you to talk normally.

- Over a period of weeks to months, work up to a level where you can briskly walk nonstop for 30 to 60 minutes without feeling winded.

- Don't count the stop-and-go casual walking you do around the house or at the office as part of your exercise program. Stop-and-go exercises don't provide significant conditioning benefits for your heart and lungs. Set aside special time for brisk, nonstop walking.

- Overweight people find that the addition of nonstop, brisk walking to their daily routines can help them lose weight without having to severely reduce their caloric intake.

- When you reach a point where you need more of a challenge, strap on a weighted backpack or add a few hills to your walking program.

- Notes on brisk-walking form: Swing your arms, take long strides, and look at the beautiful world around you.

5. Jogging

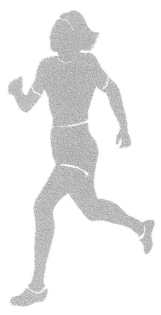

Special Advantages:

- The growing number of jogging trails and indoor/outdoor tracks make for great access and convenience. Concrete is not the best choice for a running surface (too hard), nor is grass (too bumpy).

- It's fun and motivating to jog with a companion if you like company during exercise. Pick a buddy, however, who's approximately at your level of fitness. If he/she's in much better shape, they'll run you ragged. If your companion lags far behind in speed and/or stamina, you won't be able to significantly improve your fitness.

Special Equipment Needed:

- Quality running shoes (not sneakers) are a must to protect your feet and joints from the pounding they take in jogging. Shoes should extend 3/4" beyond the longest toe, fit perfectly over athletic socks, allow no slippage of the heel, be sufficiently flexible (even when new) to be comfortable, and have shock-absorbing soles.

- Hundreds of brands and varieties of running shoes are available. Shop around until you find a perfect fit. (Athletic stores tend to have wider selections and more expert salespeople.)

- Dress in layers when it's cold; don't overdress when it's warm.

- If you have knee and/or foot problems, you may need to see an orthopedist or a podiatrist to obtain special instructions and/or an orthotic shoe insert.

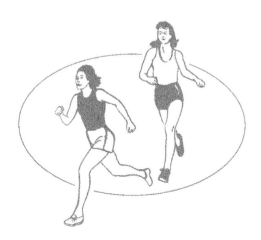

Beginning Jogging

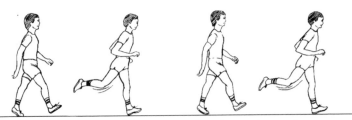

Alternate walking with slow jogging.

Advice for Beginners:
- At first, alternate walking with slow jogging, slowing to a walk whenever you reach the point where you can't talk. Gradually increase the proportion of jogging time to walking time until you are jogging on a nonstop basis. Don't expect too much too soon.

- If you feel you are able to do more, extend your time, not your speed (pace).

- Beginners should invest in a good book on jogging before beginning their program.

- Don't try to keep up with others who are in better shape than you. Exercise at your own pace.

- Take time to "warm up" and stay within your limits.
- Don't lean forward when you jog.
- Hold your forearms approximately parallel to the ground, and keep your hands and shoulders relaxed.
- Keep your strides short -- don't get your feet out ahead of your knees.
- Land on your heels, not on the balls of your feet.
- Breathe through your mouth.
- When you're within about 10 minutes of stopping jogging, begin to slow down gradually and finish by walking at a comfortable pace for several more minutes. This allows time for your circulation to clear the lactic acid from your muscles in order to avoid having them become stiff and sore.

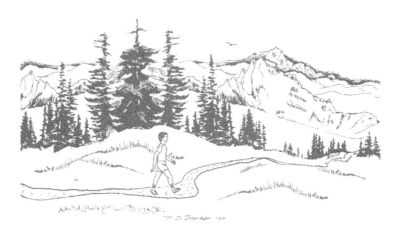

Times to Exercise

Before Breakfast

Advantages:

- Clears your mind and invigorates your body so you can begin your day with enthusiasm.
- At this refreshing time of day it's hard to make excuses for not exercising.
- You have to take a shower anyway.

Possible Disadvantages:

- It may be hard to get out of bed a little earlier.

Before Lunch

Advantages:

- Works off morning tensions.
- Refreshes you to meet the afternoon demands.
- Helps curb lunch appetite.

Possible Disadvantages:

- You've got to have a place to shower . . . or a lot of cologne.
- Your lunch break may not be long enough for you to get in an adequate exercise session and have time for lunch, too.

Before Dinner

Advantages:

- Clears the day's tensions.
- Refreshes you for evening activities.
- Helps curb dinner appetite.

Possible Disadvantages:

- Easy to find a reason not to exercise at this time of day.

Before Bed

Advantages:

- Clears your mind and helps you relax.

Possible Disadvantages:

- Easy to say -- "It's late, I'll do it tomorrow."
- Need to wait until you feel up to exercising after you've finished eating.

There are a million excuses for not exercising regularly. Here are a few:

"I don't have the time."

All it takes is a minimum of 30 minutes of aerobic exercise daily to stay in reasonable shape. "Steal" 10 minutes from your usual TV watching time, 10 minutes from your sleep time, and 10 minutes from your goof-off time, and you'll be set.

"I don't have the energy."

The vast majority of people who exercise regularly say exercise makes them "feel full of energy," and that's why they do it. Exercise, by getting the blood circulating and the muscles moving, is an ideal way to overcome frustration, relieve stress, and clear your mind of the day's problems. In this way, it serves to supply you with more energy, providing a kind of "second wind."

"I always get sore."

Sore muscles come from doing too much, too soon, and not coming to a gradual stop. Start a routine of exercise where you concentrate on gradually increasing *time* rather than speed (pace). And, before stopping, slow down gradually over 5 to 10 minutes, so your muscles won't become stiff and sore.

"It's too much work to get in shape."

A nice thing about aerobic exercise is that you can adjust the pace to suit your needs. You'll soon find the right speed that will allow you to progressively extend your exercise time to 30 minutes without becoming breathless.

"I've tried getting more exercise, but I never stick with it."

This time you will! You can afford 30 minutes of exercise every day of the week. No big deal. (If you need a motivator, exercise with a buddy, use gold stars on a calendar, or anything that works for you.) The key is to make exercise a priority and develop it into a faithful habit.

"I'm too old."

You're as old as you feel, and regular exercise will make you feel younger. Just take it slowly, and work on *gradually* increasing your muscular, cardiovascular, and respiratory endurances.

"I hate fighting the weather."

An indoor swimming pool, an exercycle, a shopping mall (for walking), and an aerobics class can help with this. If none of these suits your fancy, get a treadmill and walk *inside* on rainy days.

"I have arthritis."

Your doctor will probably recommend that you swim or cycle (indoors). Studies show that these exercises help relieve arthritic pains and stiffness.

"I'm too busy running around doing things for other people."

A half-hour of exercise every day of the week is a gift you must give yourself. It will allow you to feel and look your best, while you do more for others.

"Exercising is boring!"

Well, see what you can do to make it "fun!" Vary your walking/jogging route. Listen to music. Position your exercycle so you can watch the evening news while you pump away. Join an aerobic dance class. Exercise with a friend. Treat yourself to new athletic shoes. Challenge yourself.

"I don't know what to do with the kids."
If possible, take them with you (they need exercise, too!). Invest in an exercycle or treadmill. Many health clubs have child day care facilities; check them out.

"My family isn't interested."
That's okay. This is something you're doing for yourself.

"I'm not that interested in fitness; I've got other priorities."
Stop for a moment and reflect, "Exercise will help me live longer and better." And that's for real! And there's more.

Difficult problems often "solve themselves" while you exercise. This isn't a trick. Exercise refreshes your mind and helps you think more clearly.

"I don't have the right clothes, equipment, etc."
Buy them. It could be one of the most worthwhile investments of your life.

"I'm too fat."
So . . . you're just the one who needs exercise. Start with something easy, like walking around the block. Do that for a week. Go around twice the next week, and so on. See how much better you'll feel -- and how much less you'll want to eat! Keep at it, and you'll lose excess fat while you gain needed muscle.

"According to the charts, I'd have to jog forever just to work off one donut."

Exercise charts only tell half the story. First of all, many people find that regular aerobic exercise helps them curb their appetite. One reason for this is that exercise tends to reduce tension and depression, common causes of the "munchies." Exercise also signals the liver to convert some of its glycogen into glucose and release it into the blood, which helps curbs the appetite.

Second, regular exercise "tunes" the body and speeds its engines so they idle faster at rest. Fit people, pound per pound, burn more calories than fat people. This is because a pound of resting muscle burns more calories than a pound of fat, which is largely dormant. And, after exercising, this difference becomes even more pronounced, and this extra increase lasts for many hours.

Have faith. If you have a lot of fat to lose and are only losing 1/2-to-1 lb. per week, don't get discouraged. You're on track. Remember, the right way to lose weight is to lose excess fat gradually while you add muscle (see pages 150-151).

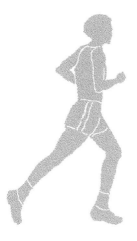

"What about *spot-reducing* exercises?"

It's true that fat tends to concentrate in specific areas of the body; it generally shows up on the hips and thighs of women, and around the waist of men.

Spot-reduction exercises like sit-ups and leg-lifts make those muscles stronger and firmer. The same fat deposits, however, still sit on top of these muscles. The fat on top of a muscle does not belong to that muscle; it belongs to the whole body. This fat will begin to "melt away" only when the demand for calories in the whole body exceeds the caloric intake.

Spot-reduction exercises don't demand a great deal of energy. Whole body aerobic exercises are better because they use large sets of muscles and require more calories to meet the increased energy requirements.

> *Note: For people who have lost some of their excess weight but still have stubborn fat stores that they don't like, selective removal of these deposits by a plastic surgery procedure called **liposuction** is possible. In this operation, the surgeon inserts a suction device through the skin and uses it to slim and contour the excessively padded areas. But, it's an **expensive way to lose weight**.*

"Is it safe to exercise if I have cardiovascular disease or have had heart surgery?"

If you have a health problem, it's important for you to check with your doctor before you make any significant changes in your schedule of physical activities.

Your physician will probably approve a moderate walking or swimming program for you. If that is the case, your doctor will start you slowly, extend the distance gradually, and then increase your speed cautiously.

Jogging and other more strenuous exercises are usually *not* recommended for those who have significant cardiovascular disease or who have had heart surgery. Walking at a pace that suits your needs is ideal. (See the F.I.T. guidelines given on pages 156-157 and follow your doctor's advice.)

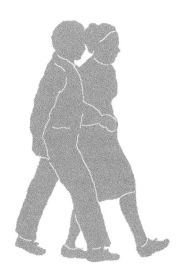

Stress

Stress is the summation of all our emotional, mental, and physical responses to the threatening inner and outer conflicts that challenge us everyday. While some stress helps us stay sharp and responsive, too much stress is destructive. This turbulent state causes us to become tense, irritable, apprehensive, and frightened. Stress causes the adrenal glands to make and release a flood of adrenalin which makes our pulse race, blood pressure climb, heart work harder, and platelets become stickier. These changes can cause a heart attack. To stay out of this danger zone may require that we gain a greater understanding of ourselves, change our attitudes and goals, and obtain better control of our responses to the seemingly adverse situations that appear to surround and confront us. But how to do this?

Difficulty in maintaining a suitable balance between our past, present, and future in this incredible age of discovery, change, and turmoil can become a source of unbearable tension for any of us.

We need balance in our lives because otherwise we may live too much in the future or too much in the past. Although we must learn from the past to plan for the future and be inspired by what is yet to come, our focal point should be the ever present now, because that's the reality of life.

The best defense against developing excessive stress in response to the many challenges in our lives is to maintain a happy, relaxed mental state by doing God's work in the here and now to the best of our ability. This can be done most successfully by helping those who need us in a spirit of love. When we do this, God rewards us with a joyful life free of anxiety, fear, and worry.

Being kind, thoughtful, and generous to others is the surest way for any of us to find peace and happiness. Since we all yearn for this mental state, why not go for it by following this "can't miss" plan?

This plan for peace of mind, serenity of soul, and exhilaration of spirit could be more effective than the billions of dollars spent yearly in the United States on tranquilizers and sedatives to combat fear, loneliness, and simple depression. And not only would we be happier people, our homes, cities, states, nation, and world would also be better.

Time passes very quickly, and life here is over almost before we know it. We can find great happiness in our earthly days and defuse the anxiety in our lives if we follow the late, beloved *Mother Teresa's advice* and serve those in need with love and joy in our hearts as we travel our personal roads to eternity.

There is infinite wisdom in the *universal prayer of St. Francis* (page 262). You may wish to memorize it. The simple repetition of this prayer each day can bring greater peace and joy to all who do so.

Section IV:

Simplified Program

A Simplified Program for Heart-Healthy Living

General Considerations 183-184

The Five Cardinal Rules for
  Heart-Healthy Living 184-187

Three Additional Strategies 188-191

    1. Take Antioxidant Vitamins 188-189

    2. Reduce the Stickiness of
       Your Platelets if They Are
       Too Sticky 189-190

    3. Select a Good Doctor and
       Follow His or Her Advice 191

General Considerations

Heart attack and stroke are the leading killers in the industrial world. But the good news is that the death rate for cardiovascular disease in the U.S. has decreased about 20% in recent years due to increased prevention and treatment efforts. Now we must go the *rest of the way.*

Hardening of the arteries (atherosclerosis) starts early in life. Autopsy examinations of adolescent American accident victims show that most already have fatty plaques in their coronary arteries. These findings indicate that we must start in childhood to prevent heart disease from developing. This could be done by teaching the children of today the rules of heart-healthy living in three interrelated ways:

1. Good example and instruction by parents in the home.
2. Positive guidance by pediatricians and family physicians.
3. Proper training by teachers in the schools.

"An ounce of *prevention* early on is worth a pound of *cure* in later years." But prevention efforts must be both simple and effective if they are to be widely adopted.

Our guidelines pass this test . . . they are *simple* and *effective.* Avoid smoking. Eat a proper diet. Get regular aerobic exercise. Attain and maintain a healthful weight. Control stress.

These guidelines should be followed throughout life. They can help healthy people avoid premature hardening of their arteries, and they can also keep cardiovascular disease, if present, from progressing.

This is especially important for patients who need surgery for the complications of atherosclerosis. This is because surgery is only a *mechanical* solution to a structural problem, and this solution fails to address the underlying *biochemical causes* of the problem.

Given adequate time, all arteries would eventually wear out. In earlier years so many people died of infections (such as smallpox, pneumonia, typhoid, diphtheria, tuberculosis, staph infections, strep infections, meningitis, and appendicitis) that few lived long enough for this to happen. In fact, most people died before reaching age 50.

Now that we are living longer . . . the average life span in the U.S. is about 72 years for men and 78 for women . . . nearly *half* of us will die from hardened arteries and clots unless we take steps now to prevent this from happening later.

The Five Cardinal Rules
for
Heart-Healthy Living

To increase our chances of living to a ripe old age with our mental faculties and physical capabilities in top form, it's necessary to follow an effective plan to keep our arteries in good condition. Our plan may be expressed through the letters: **S** . . . **D-E-W** . . . **S** which identify the core subjects of the five cardinal rules for heart-healthy living:

Smoking . . . **D**iet-**E**xercise-**W**eight . . . **S**tress.

The prime objective of this program is to prevent the development of atherosclerosis which causes clots to form that block the flow channel of vital arteries (Figs. 33-34, pp. 74-75).

This program works in two main ways. *First,* it acts to correct the biochemical causes of atherosclerosis by lowering the blood levels of homocysteine, LDL cholesterol, and triglycerides while elevating that of HDL cholesterol. *Second,* the program acts to decrease the ability of blood to clot by lowering the level of fibrinogen and by keeping platelets from becoming sticky. The cardinal rules are:

Smoking • Don't smoke, even passively.

Diet • Eat a delicious low-saturated fat, high fiber, low-*trans* fatty acid, low-sugar, proper calorie diet that includes non/low-fat dairy products.

The **Better Life Diet**© (pages 136-151) reflects the general admonition that if it grows in the ground, grows on trees, isn't refined, swims, or has feathers, it's O.K. But if you have a genetic "cholesterol problem," you may need the more restrictive Pritikin or Ornish diets.

Exercise • Accumulate at least 30 minutes of moderate activity every day.

Weight • Attain and maintain the weight at which you both feel and look your best.

Stress • Strive for an inner peace that allows you to accept problems as a natural part of life. This mental attitude is best attained by helping others in a spirit of love.

Rules for Heart-Healthy Living

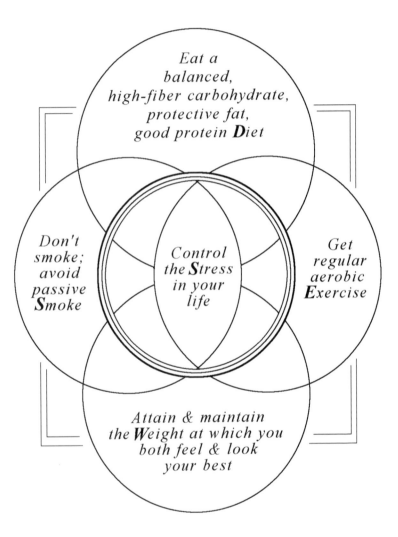

Eat a
balanced,
high-fiber carbohydrate,
protective fat,
good protein **D**iet

Don't
smoke;
avoid
passive
Smoke

Control
the **S**tress
in your
life

Get
regular
aerobic
Exercise

Attain & maintain
the **W**eight at which you
both feel & look
your best

*Figure 59 - The five interlocking rules for heart-healthy living
are vital to good health and long life.*

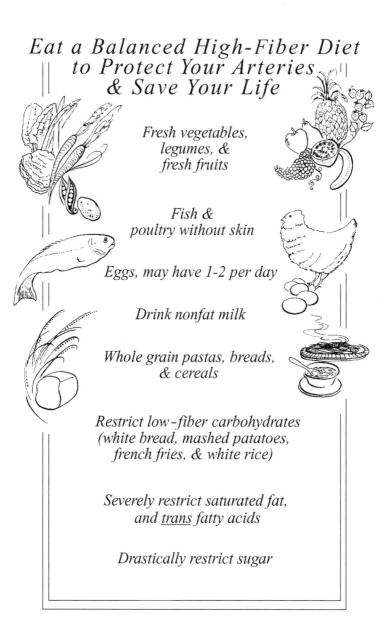

Eat a Balanced High-Fiber Diet to Protect Your Arteries & Save Your Life

Fresh vegetables,
legumes, &
fresh fruits

Fish &
poultry without skin

Eggs, may have 1-2 per day

Drink nonfat milk

Whole grain pastas, breads,
& cereals

Restrict low-fiber carbohydrates
(white bread, mashed patatoes,
french fries, & white rice)

Severely restrict saturated fat,
and <u>trans</u> fatty acids

Drastically restrict sugar

*Figure 60 - **The Better Life Diet**:©*
Tasty meals that are good for you.

Three Additional Strategies

If the majority of people in the United States would follow the five cardinal rules for heart-healthy living, the incidence of atherosclerosis would dramatically decrease within two decades. Some people need more. These are the people who have a family or personal history of heart or artery disease and/or have one or more of the following abnormal blood chemistries:

1. An HDL cholesterol level below 30 mg/dL in men and below 40 mg/dL in women. (HDL cholesterol transports LDL cholesterol and probably other fats out of the arterial wall and out of the lipid core of soft plaques.)

2. A fasting triglyceride level above 200 mg/dL. (Triglycerides are fats derived both from the fatty foods in our diet, and from conversion of excess carbohydrates and proteins into fat.)

3. An LDL cholesterol level above 150 mg/dL. The *ideal* value for this lipid is under 100 mg/dL.

4. A fibrinogen level above 350 mg/dL. (Fibrinogen is the blood protein that forms clots.)

5. A fasting platelet aggregation score above 30. (Sticky platelets cause blood to clot.)

6. Elevated levels of homocysteine (see next page).

These people need the following three *additional strategies:*

1. Take Antioxidant Vitamins

"Free oxygen radical" is a popular term that is currently used to explain nearly everything that goes wrong in the body, from cancer to heart disease and from arthritis to cataracts. This term refers to an oxygen-bearing chemical which has a deficiency of electrons in the outer orbit of its oxygen atoms. These electron-deficient atoms severely damage neighboring atoms by robbing them of their electrons.

A current theory suggests that low-density lipoprotein cholesterol (LDL) damages the inner portion of the arterial wall only when it becomes *oxidized* and has free oxygen radicals. If this is proven to be true, it could explain why heart attacks occur in some patients with low LDL cholesterol, but not in others with high LDL cholesterol.

But there is *good* news. In addition to enjoying a healthy, nutritious diet, you can further protect yourself against free oxygen radicals by taking 50 mg of Vitamin B6, 500 mg of Vitamin C, and 400 units of Vitamin E daily. And these vitamins only cost about 12 cents a day. We also advise taking a good multivitamin that contains 0.4 mg of folic acid daily. In addition, we suggest that people with multiple risk factors also take 30 mg of coenzyme Q-10 daily. This powerful antioxidant costs about 50 cents a day.

A further benefit of taking Vitamin B6 and folic acid is that these agents (and Vitamin B12) reduce the blood level of *homocysteine,* an amino acid, which in high concentration injures endothelial cells and predisposes the inner arterial wall to develop atherosclerosis. Smoking, inactivity, and other factors that cause atherosclerosis also increase homocysteine.

2. Reduce the Stickiness of Your Platelets If They Are Too Sticky

The degree of stickiness that platelets can develop is unique to each person. Platelets that become *very sticky* can cause fatal blood clots. Such platelets may *adhere, activate,* and *aggregate* on the diseased flow surface of hardened (atherosclerotic) arteries, especially when soft plaques rupture and release their deadly lipid contents. These platelet aggregates may cause clots to form which can block the channel and stop the flow of blood to vital regions of our bodies. Such lack of blood supply causes heart attacks, strokes, high blood pressure, impaired walking ability, and gangrene of the feet and lower legs.

Life depends on an almost endless series of checks and balances of which the stickiness of our platelets is but one example. If our platelets couldn't stick together, we would *bleed to death.* But if they are too sticky, we would *clot to death.* What we want is the right balance.

Millions of people take an aspirin a day to reduce the stickiness of their platelets even though they don't know whether this is either necessary or effective for them. Studies at **The Hope Heart Institute** in Seattle, Washington, have shown that about 25% of people don't need aspirin because their platelets aren't sticky. The other 75% of people have sticky platelets. About 2/3 of these people have platelets that respond adequately to aspirin and 1/3 do not.

The only way to find out who needs treatment to control excessive platelet aggregation and with what medication is to *do an appropriate test.* Few laboratories do this test. **The Hope Heart Institute** research staff has developed an automated method that could make this measurement widely available in the future.

3. Select a Good Doctor and Follow His or Her Advice

If your physician finds that you have a "gene" problem, he/she may advise the Pritikin or the Ornish diet.

If you are retaining fluid or have high blood pressure, your physician may request you to restrict salt. It's easy to take too much salt since about 90% of what we consume is already in our food. Packaged, canned, and fast foods contain by far the most salt. Read the labels.

In addition, your physician may find that you need medications to decrease your blood pressure; decrease your blood levels of homocysteine, LDL cholesterol, triglycerides, and sugar; increase your blood level of HDL cholesterol; and regulate other chemistries.

Also, you may need *magnesium* since most people are deficient in this essential mineral that steadies and strengthens the heart beat.

Further, if you are a woman who has passed through menopause, your physician may advise you to take estrogen replacement therapy to help reduce your risk of developing coronary heart disease, osteoporosis, and possibly Alzheimer's disease.

While medications are *not* a substitute for the five cardinal rules and the three additional strategies for heart-healthy living, they can be very important.

Section V:
Surgical Procedures

Surgical Procedures for Arteries Irreversibly Damaged by Atherosclerosis and its Complications

Two Types of Operations:
Vascular and Endovascular 194-203

Surgery to Increase the Blood Supply
to the _Heart_ 204-219

- Balloon Angioplasty for Single Coronary
  Obstruction 206
- Balloon Angioplasty with
  Stent Placement 207
- Single Coronary Bypass
  Using an Internal Mammary Artery 208
- Balloon Angioplasty for
  Double Coronary Obstruction 209
- Double Coronary Bypass
  Using Saphenous Vein Grafts 210
- Double Coronary Bypass Using
  Internal Mammary Artery Grafts 211
- Triple Coronary Bypass
  Using Saphenous Vein Grafts 212
- Quadruple Coronary Bypass
  Using Saphenous Vein Grafts 213
- Quadruple Coronary Bypass Using
  Three Saphenous Vein Grafts and One
  Internal Mammary Artery Graft 214
- Quintuple Coronary Bypass Using
  Both Internal Mammary Arteries 215
- Combined Coronary Bypass and
  Heart Valve Surgery 216-219

**Surgery to Increase the Blood Supply
to the _Brain_ and to Prevent Embolic
Obstruction of Flow** 220-221
- Carotid Endarterectomy 221

**Surgery to Increase the Blood Supply
to the _Kidneys_** 222-224
- Balloon Angioplasty and
  Stent Placement to Correct Narrowing
  of a Renal Artery.................................. 223
- Bypass Grafts to Renal Arteries 224

**Surgery to Increase the
Blood Flow to the _Legs_** 225-239
- Aortobifemoral Bypass 228
- Femorofemoral Bypass 229
- Axillofemoral Bypass 230
- Combined Axillofemoral
  and Femorofemoral Bypass 231
- Balloon Angioplasty of
  Left Common Iliac Artery........................ 232
- Endarterectomy of the Arteries
  at the Groin.. 233
- Nature's "Operation".. 234
- Balloon Angioplasty and
  Stent Placement of Distal
  Superficial Femoral Artery............................ 235
- Above-Knee Femoropopliteal
  Bypass (Synthetic Graft) 236
- Below-Knee Femoropopliteal
  Bypass (Vein Graft) 237
- Femorotibial Bypass (Vein Graft) 238
- Femoropedal Bypass (Vein Graft)................ 239

Surgery for _Aortic Aneurysms_ 240-241
- Graft for Thoracic Aneurysm 240
- Graft for Abdominal Aneurysm 241

193

Two Types of Operations

The need for surgery to treat the complications of atherosclerosis is an admission that prevention has failed either because no program was followed, the program followed was inadequate, or the program was started too late. Whatever the reason, surgery is a vital backup for these patients. For optimal results, the best of surgical and medical care must be combined.

While surgery can literally accomplish wonders, we must not forget that all who are at risk to develop atherosclerosis and related clot formation need the preventive measures discussed in Sections III and IV. The "all who are at risk" includes most everyone in our affluent society. If the rules for heart-healthy living were followed, far fewer people would need operative help.

There are two very different types of operations that can be used to treat the abnormalities that occur in arteries as a result of atherosclerosis and clot formation. The first type is classified as "**open**" and the second as "**closed**."

The open type, called *vascular surgery*, exposes the arteries from the outside. For the most part, this type of surgery involves endarterectomy procedures (Fig. 61), bypass grafts (Fig. 62), and replacement grafts (Fig. 63).

The closed type, called *endovascular surgery*, is done from inside the artery with devices brought to the diseased areas by long, slender, hollow tubes called catheters that are inserted through the skin into the arterial system with only a needle puncture. This new type of surgery is evolving rapidly.

Vascular Surgery

Vascular surgery operations in general use today have been proven by time to be safe and reliable. Operations of this type are performed in well-lighted operating rooms by surgeons who make incisions through the skin and underlying tissues to expose the artery. The operations for obstructions usually involve opening the artery and removing the material that is blocking the vessel, a procedure called *endarterectomy,* or establishing a new pathway for blood to flow around the site of the blockage, a procedure called *bypass graft placement.* The operation for aneurysms usually involves creating a secure channel inside the aneurysm for passage of blood, a procedure called *replacement graft insertion.*

Bypass Grafts for Obstructions

This procedure is accomplished by suturing one end of a graft to an opening in the wall of the artery above the blockage and the other end to an opening in the wall of the artery below the obstruction. The blood flows from the artery above the block through the graft into the artery below the obstruction and from there it flows on to the tissues to supply their needs.

Replacement Grafts for Aneurysms

The surgeon clamps the artery, usually the aorta, above and below the aneurysm, opens its front wall, removes the clot and debris, and then sutures a plastic graft to the inside of the aorta (artery) above and below the ballooned-out region to establish a safe channel with walls that won't rupture. The surgeon then trims the aneurysm sac and sutures its edges together to tightly encircle the artificial graft with a layer of living tissue.

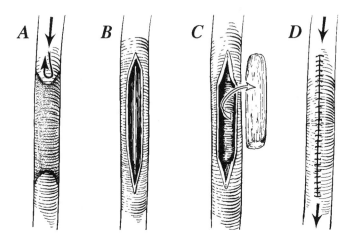

Figure 61 - Increasing the flow of red blood to the tissues by an endarterectomy procedure involves cutting into the artery, removing the material that is blocking the flow channel, and suturing the remaining wall back together.

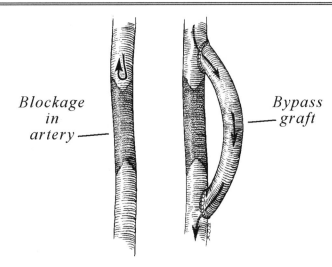

Figure 62 - Increasing the flow of red blood to the tissues by a bypass graft involves suturing one end of the graft to an opening made in the artery above the blockage and the other end to an opening made below the blockage.

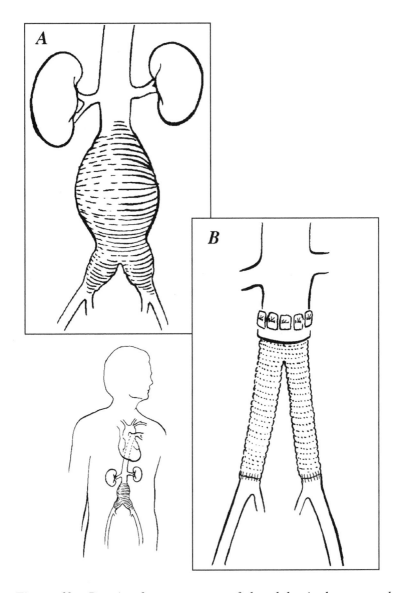

Figure 63 - Repair of an aneurysm of the abdominal aorta and common iliac arteries with a bifurcated Dacron graft to convey red blood to pelvis and legs. Wrapping of this replacement graft by the outer layer of the aneurysm wall is not shown.

Endovascular Surgery

Endovascular surgical operations are procedures performed from within the blood channel with catheters inserted over guide wires into the flow channel of arteries, usually distant from the sites of blockage which require treatment. These catheters are advanced to the blocked areas under the continuous x-ray visualization provided by monitor screens.

Some catheters have *inflatable balloons, cutting instruments,* or *grinding burrs* at their tips that are used to remove the obstructions. These operations are carried out in the semidarkness of space-age procedure rooms by cardiologists, interventional radiologists, or vascular surgeons who visualize what is happening deep inside the body on the x-ray monitor screens.

The operator begins these inside-the-artery operations by puncturing the skin, usually at the groin, with a needle that is advanced inward through the front wall of the underlying artery to enter the flow channel. The operator then passes a guide wire through the needle into the artery and advances it upward or downward depending on the direction that the needle was inserted.

The operator then withdraws the needle, leaving the guide wire in place, and inserts a relatively large but short catheter, called a *sheath,* over the guide wire and advances it into the artery. The sheath has a *diaphragm* at its entrance through which guide wires and catheters can be introduced, withdrawn, and replaced without loss of blood. The sheath is like an on-off-ramp to a superhighway.

When the operator has properly positioned a catheter, he/she withdraws the guide wire and advances the catheter

Passage of Catheters into Arteries

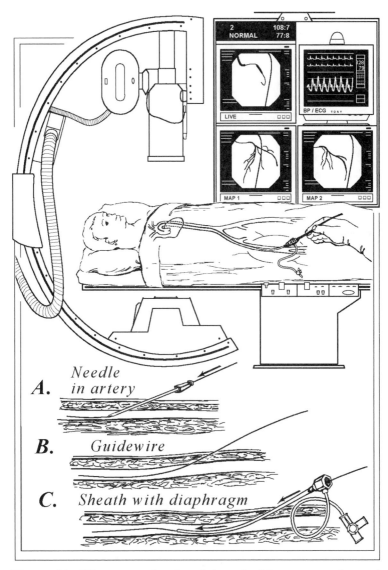

Figure 64 - Placement of a sheath into the big artery at the groin quickly establishes access into the arterial system and allows guide wires and smaller catheters to be inserted, removed, and reinserted easily without loss of blood.

to the desired location, such as into the coronary arteries. Next, the operator performs arteriograms by injecting dye and taking films at a rapid rate to provide a motion picture sequence -- "an x-ray movie" -- of the flow of this fluid through the vessels.

In the case of a coronary artery, if an area of marked narrowing is discovered, the cardiologist passes a slender guide wire with a very fine, flexible tip through the inserting catheter. The tip of this guide wire is so flexible that if it is pushed into the wall, the tip will fold back on itself and produce no injury.

The cardiologist passes this fine guide wire through the site of narrowing and then advances a balloon-tipped catheter over it to center the deflated balloon across this site.

After checking to make sure that all is ready, the cardiologist inflates the balloon to high pressures that stretch and compress the wall and enlarge the lumen at the site of narrowing, a procedure called *Percutaneous Transluminal Coronary Angioplasty (PTCA* - page 202).

If the balloon result isn't good, the operator may repeat the procedure or advance a catheter with a burr or cutting device at its tip and grind or shave the obstruction away.

These balloon and other type procedures may tear the inner wall and partially detach a portion of it. If the fragment faces into the current, the flow force will drive it into the channel and block the blood path. To correct this problem, an ingenious expandable wire mesh device, called the *endovascular stent* , has been developed (page 203).

To deploy a stent, the operator passes a balloon-tipped

catheter that has a *contracted* stent positioned *over* the *deflated* balloon. The operator advances this catheter over the guide wire which had been had left in place after the initial dilation procedure.

In the case of a disrupted coronary artery, the cardiologist positions the balloon/stent across the site of blockage and inflates the balloon which *expands* the stent. The expanded wire mesh compresses the separated layers of the coronary artery wall back together and *restores* an enlarged flow channel. The cardiologist then deflates the balloon and withdraws it, leaving the expanded stent which *maintains* the channel. The use of stents has extended the successful use of balloon angioplasty in the coronary arteries and elsewhere in the arterial system for the treatment of obstructions due to atherosclerosis and clot formations.

Endovascular techniques are being developed for placing grafts inside of aneurysms to bridge or span the dilated areas. Few aneurysms can be safely taken care of by this technique at the present time. Further developments, however, may be anticipated in this advancing field which will expand the use of endovascular grafts for patients with aneurysms.

Vascular and endovascular surgeons can now treat properly selected patients afflicted by diseased arteries caused by atherosclerosis and clots with relative safety and great benefit. Despite these remarkable advances, **our emphasis must remain on** *decreasing the need for operations of any type.* This can be accomplished for most patients by heart-healthy living begun at an early age and continued thereafter. Such a program would go a long way toward preventing atherosclerosis and its complications of blockage and aneurysm formation from developing as we age.

Balloon Angioplasty

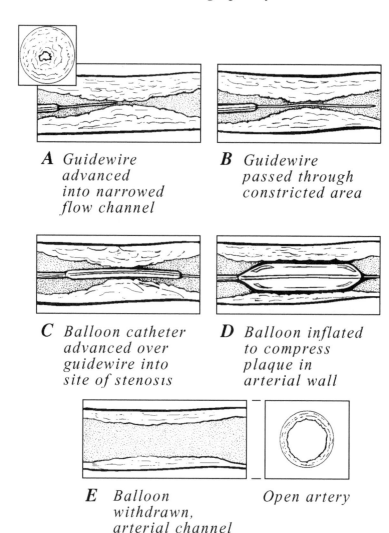

A Guidewire
advanced
into narrowed
flow channel

B Guidewire
passed through
constricted area

C Balloon catheter
advanced over
guidewire into
site of stenosis

D Balloon inflated
to compress
plaque in
arterial wall

E Balloon
withdrawn,
arterial channel
enlarged

Open artery

Figure 65 - Balloon angioplasty is an endovascular operation that
enlarges the narrowed flow channel of an atherosclerotic artery by
inflating a balloon to dilate the obstructed site.

Placement of Stent

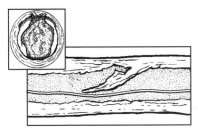

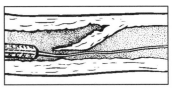

A *Detached portion of arterial wall blocks channel*

B *Deflated balloon with contracted stent advanced over guidewire*

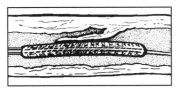

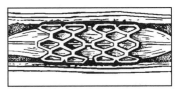

C *Balloon catheter with stent moved into place*

D *Balloon inflated, stent expanded, wall restored*

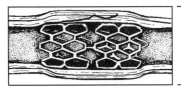

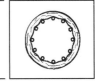

E *Deflated balloon removed leaving stent in place*

Open artery

Figure 66 - Balloon angioplasty complicated by blockage of the flow channel due to partial detachment of a portion of the wall. This complication is corrected by expanding a contracted wire mesh stent that compresses the separated layers back together and restores an enlarged flow channel.

Surgery to Increase the
Blood Supply to the Heart Muscle

Last year about *900,000* operations were performed in the
United States to increase the blood supply to the heart muscle
at a cost of approximately $20 billion. About half of these
operations were closed (endovascular) procedures performed
by cardiologists using catheters with balloons or other
devices, while the other half were performed by surgeons
using open-heart techniques to place bypass grafts.

In general, *endovascular surgery* is best used for patients
who have severe but localized disease of only one or two
coronary vessels, while *vascular surgery* is best used to
implant as many bypass grafts as needed for patients with
severe disease of all their main coronary arteries.

The main advantages of the balloon procedures are that they
require only a needle puncture, and the patients recover much
faster than after open-heart operations. But there are two
disadvantages, *acute closure* and *recurrent narrowing*.

Prior to the use of stents, acute closure developed in 3-4% of
patients. Now, with the use of stents, the frequency of this
complication has been reduced to about 1%. When it occurs,
most of the patients must be rushed to the operating room for
placement of bypass grafts.

Prior to the use of stents, severe narrowing recurred after 3 to
6 months at the site of the balloon dilation in about 33% of
the patients undergoing this procedure. With stents, this
complication has been reduced to about 15%. Most patients
who develop recurrent stenoses (narrowings) will require
additional procedures, some repeat balloon dilations and
others bypass grafts. Research continues in this area.

Surgeons most frequently use segments of the largest superficial vein in the leg to bypass blocked coronary arteries. About 50%, however, of these greater saphenous grafts develop severe atherosclerosis after 7 to 10 years and close off.

Atherosclerosis rarely develops in the delicate internal mammary arteries that lie one on each side of the breastbone inside the front of the chest. When these vessels are used for coronary bypass, the results are outstandingly good: about 95% of the grafts are open and functioning well after 10 years with no evidence of disease in their walls.

Because of these results, heart surgeons are now using mammary grafts frequently, including using them in "mini" operations to bypass blockages of the anterior descending branch of the left coronary artery. Patients recover more quickly from these smaller operations done through short incisions without the use of the heart-lung machine.

The delicate gastroepiploic artery, which runs along the lower border of the stomach, also works very well as a graft to bypass obstructions of the coronary arteries.

The risk of mortality today for patients in good condition who must undergo either balloon angioplasty or bypass grafts for blockages of their coronary arteries should not exceed 1%.

The main drawback of standard bypass surgery done with the heart-lung machine is that most patients need to convalesce for 6 to 8 weeks before they can return to full activity. But a strong recommendation for the bypass procedure is that even if the upper portions of all the coronary vessels are severely blocked, excellent results maybe anticipated for many years in 90% of these patients.

Balloon Angioplasty for
Single Right Coronary Obstruction

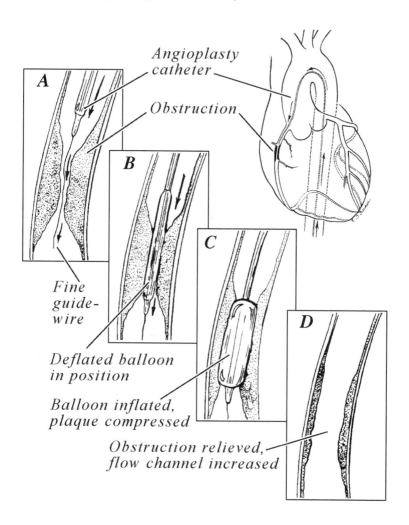

Angioplasty
catheter

Obstruction

A

B

C

D

Fine
guide-
wire

Deflated balloon
in position

Balloon inflated,
plaque compressed

Obstruction relieved,
flow channel increased

Figure 67 - Balloon angioplasty for severe stenosis (narrowing) of the upper mid-right coronary artery. This is the procedure of choice for most single and many double coronary artery blockages.

Balloon Angioplasty with Stent Placement

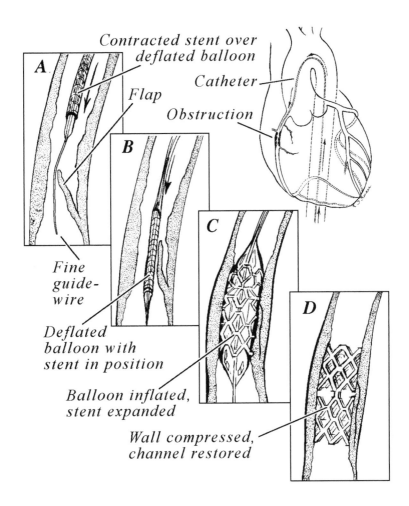

Figure 68 - Use of wire mesh stent with balloon angioplasty for severe stenosis of the upper mid-right coronary artery. When balloon angioplasty partially detaches a segment of the wall, the dangling fragment will obstruct the flow channel if it faces into the current. Should this happen, use of a stent forces the layers of the wall back together and restores an enlarged channel which converts a balloon failure into a success.

Single Coronary Bypass Using an
Internal Mammary Artery Graft
from Inside the Chest

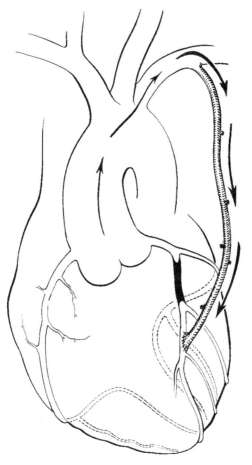

Figure 69 - Use of the left internal mammary artery to bring a new supply of red blood to the front of the heart when the upper anterior descending branch of the left coronary is completely blocked. This blockage is difficult to treat successfully by balloon angioplasty. In contrast, an internal mammary graft may be counted on to stay open indefinitely in this location under these circumstances. Branches of graft are closed by clips or cautery.

Balloon Angioplasty for
Double Coronary Obstruction,
One With and One Without a Stent

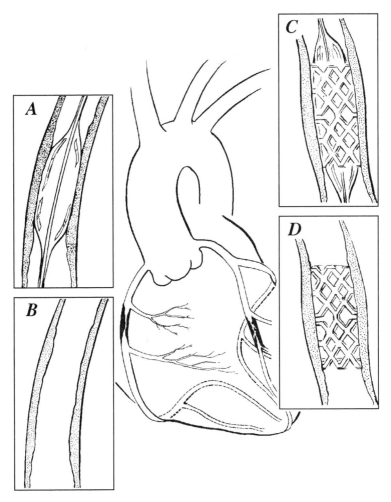

Figure 70 - Use of balloon angioplasty alone for an area of severe stenosis of the upper mid-right coronary artery, and use of balloon angioplasty with stent placement for severe stenosis of the upper midportion of the anterior descending branch of the left coronary artery.

Double Coronary Bypass Using
Saphenous Vein Grafts
from the Legs

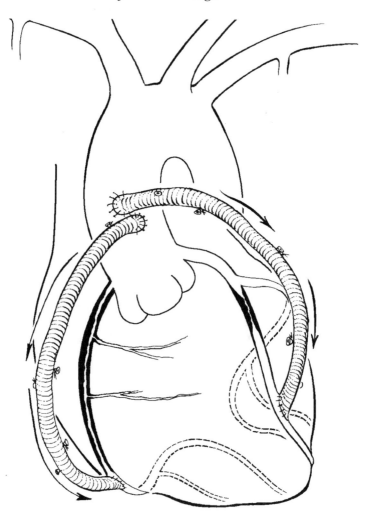

Figure 71 - Placement of two saphenous bypass grafts (superficial leg veins) from the aorta to the open coronary arteries beyond the severe obstructions brings new sources of red blood to supply the impoverished heart muscle. Branches of vein are tied off.

Double Coronary Bypass Using
Both Internal Mammary Grafts

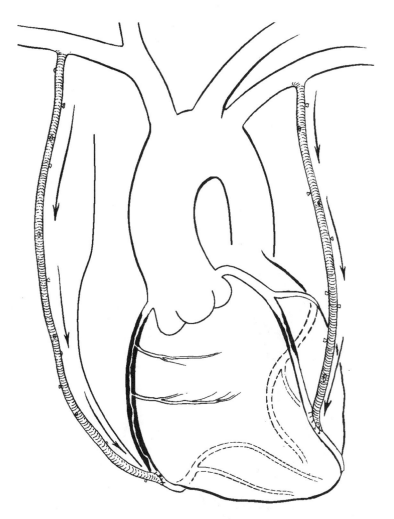

Figure 72 - Use of both internal mammary arteries to convey red blood to the same two coronary sites, as shown in the previous figure, bypassing the areas of blockage. The advantage of using the internal mammaries is that they last longer than saphenous vein grafts; the disadvantage is that they are more difficult to use.

Triple Coronary Bypass Using
Saphenous Grafts

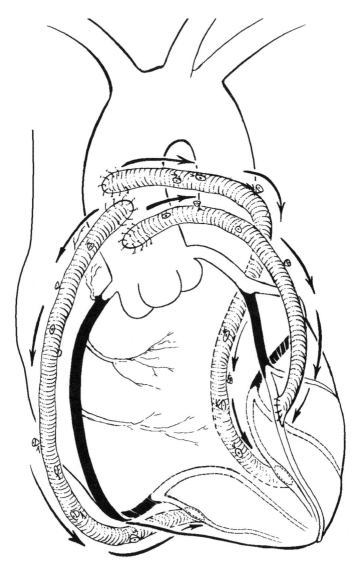

*Figure 73 - Use of three saphenous vein grafts to convey red blood
to three coronary sites, bypassing the areas of severe blockage.*

Quadruple Coronary Bypass Using Saphenous Grafts

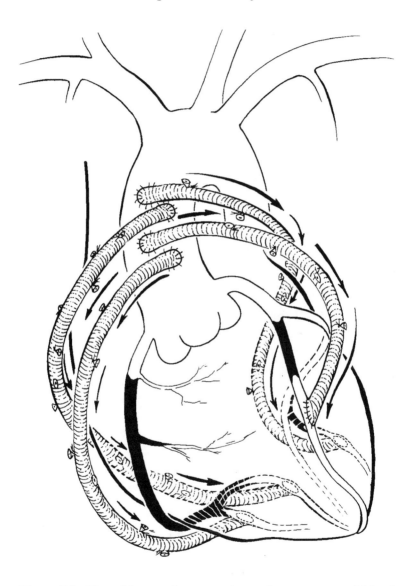

Figure 74 - Use of four saphenous vein grafts to convey red blood to four coronary sites, bypassing the areas of severe blockage.

Quadruple Coronary Bypass Using Three Saphenous Grafts and One Internal Mammary Artery Graft

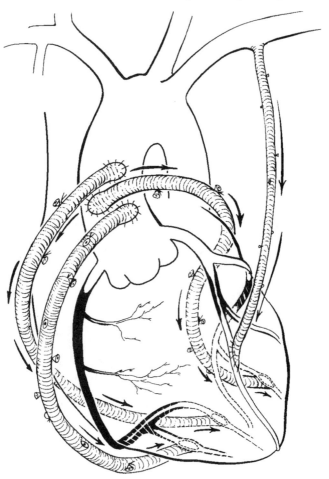

Figure 75 - Use of three saphenous vein grafts and the left internal mammary artery to convey red blood to four coronary sites, bypassing the areas of severe blockage. The left internal mammary is used for the most important vessel, the anterior descending branch of the left coronary. This bypass strategy is used frequently today.

Quintuple Coronary Bypass Using
Both Internal Mammary Arteries

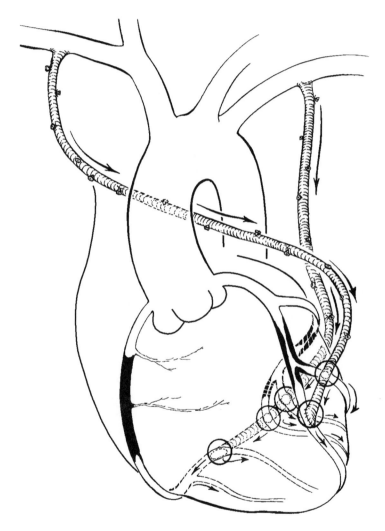

Figure 76 - Use of both internal mammary arteries to convey red blood to five coronary sites (circled), bypassing areas of severe blockage. This procedure is technically difficult, but it gives excellent long-term results.

Heart Valve Repair or Replacement in Conjunction With Surgery to Increase the Blood Supply to the Heart

A considerable number of older patients who require surgery to increase the blood supply to their hearts also need to have the function of their aortic and/or mitral valves improved. If either of these valves are too small or leak (or both), the heart is in increased trouble. To pump the same volume of blood, the heart has to work harder when the valves don't work right. It's like a motor with gears grinding that is running out of gas. When both problems are fixed . . . more fuel and well-functioning gears . . . the motor hums. The heart is the same.

When our natural heart valves are functioning properly, they are a marvel of efficiency, moving swiftly in response to the pressure of the blood to open and close. Valves may become stiff and hard. When this happens, the diseased valve obstructs the flow of blood and forces the heart to do more pressure work. If valves leak, the heart has to do more volume work.

The most frequent mitral valve problem associated with decreased blood supply to the heart is leakage. The decision to repair or replace the valve is made by the surgeon at the time of operation.

The most frequent aortic valve problem associated with decreased blood supply is narrowing of the valve. The cusps of the aortic valve may become thick, stiff, and even rigid due to calcification. Such valves may also leak because their rigid cusps can't close. In other patients, the problem may be purely leakage. When aortic valve surgery is required, the valve must nearly always be replaced because effective repair procedures are seldom possible.

There are several different types of valves that heart surgeons can use to replace their patients' diseased valves. Many are made of plastic and metal. Some are pig valves and others are human valves obtained from recently deceased accident victims.

In addition, in young patients the surgeon may replace the patient's diseased aortic valve with their own normal pulmonary valve and replace that valve with one removed from a recently deceased accident victim. This complex operation was developed by Dr. Donald Ross in England 30 years ago, and his first patient is still doing well.

Animal valves and valves made from other animal tissues are treated with chemicals to make them durable, flexible, and resistant to clot formation.

Because artificial (mechanical) valves are constructed of metal and plastic components, they tend to last longer than processed animal valves. But mechanical valves are more prone to have clots form on them than are tissue valves. Pieces of these clots may break off and be carried by the blood to the brain where they can produce a major stroke.

Clot formation can also impair the valve's function and necessitate emergency reoperation. Because of this, patients with mechanical valves are given drugs (usually Coumadin) to decrease the blood's ability to clot. Frequently, this is not required for patients with tissue valves, especially those from humans.

Single Coronary Bypass and Aortic Valve Replacement

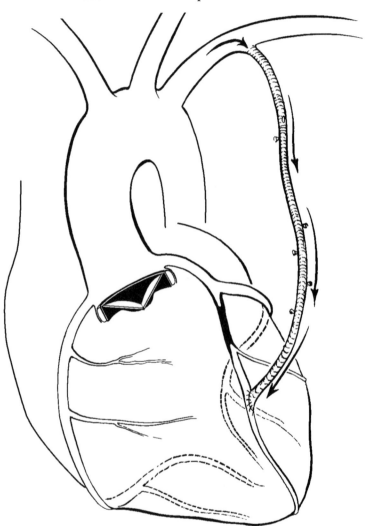

Figure 77 - Combined single coronary bypass using the left internal mammary artery to carry red blood to the anterior descending branch of the left coronary artery and aortic valve replacement with a St. Jude artificial heart valve (valve in closed position shown in cross section).

Double Coronary Bypass and Double Valve Replacement

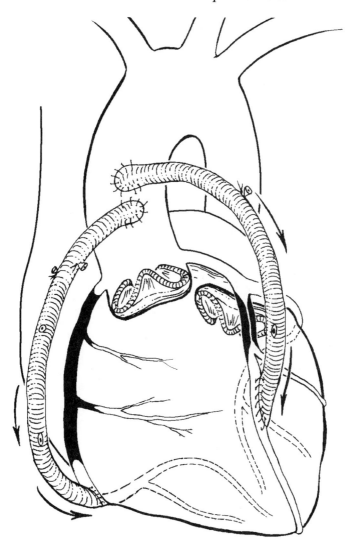

Figure 78 - Combined double coronary bypass (right and anterior descending branch of left) using two saphenous vein grafts and double valve replacement (aortic and mitral) with chemically processed pig valves.

Surgery to Increase
the Blood Supply to the Brain
and to Prevent
Embolic Obstruction of Flow

Carotid endarterectomy is the second most frequent arterial operation; the coronary bypass procedure is the most common.

Approximately 100,000 patients undergo carotid surgery each year in the United States for the purpose of preventing strokes. By far the most frequent operation performed for this purpose is carotid endarterectomy, a procedure in which the surgeon removes the obstruction(s) and/or area(s) of ulceration that involve the division point (bifurcation) of the common carotid artery and the first portions (seldom over an inch) of the internal and external carotid arteries.

Today, patients undergoing this type of surgery are usually in the hospital for less than 24 hours, in contrast to a few years ago when the average stay was 5 to 6 days. This shortened stay reduces the yearly health care costs for carotid surgery in the United States by about $300,000,000.

Carotid Endarterectomy

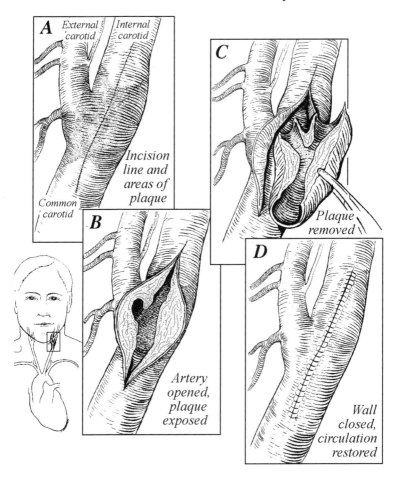

Figure 79 - The surgeon opens the obstructed division point of the common carotid artery, removes the diseased inner wall and any clot that is blocking the flow channel (the endarterectomy procedure), and sutures the outer wall back together to restore a full-caliber pathway with a smooth, glistening, clot resistant surface for the passage of red blood to the brain. This operation has been proven to be safe, effective, and long-lasting. Endovascular procedures have also been developed for this purpose, but cannot be recommended for general use at this time.

Surgery to Increase the Blood
Supply to the Kidneys

The vascular surgeon can restore a full supply of red blood to a kidney that has a blocked artery either by an endarterectomy or a bypass graft procedure.

Because endovascular renal (kidney) artery surgery is quicker and less invasive than open vascular surgery, this relatively new technique has become the procedure of choice for the initial treatment of renal artery blockage. Interventional radiologists perform most of these procedures.

The radiologist dilates the site of blockage in the renal artery with a balloon, places a stent (if necessary) to help keep the enlarged channel open, and then sends the patient home a few hours later. Recurrent stenosis (narrowing), as in the coronaries, is the main complication and occurs with about the same frequency.

If blockage recurs, another endovascular procedure will usually be performed. If the blockage recurs again, placement of a bypass graft by a vascular surgeon may be necessary.

Balloon Angioplasty and Stent Placement to Correct Narrowing of a Renal Artery

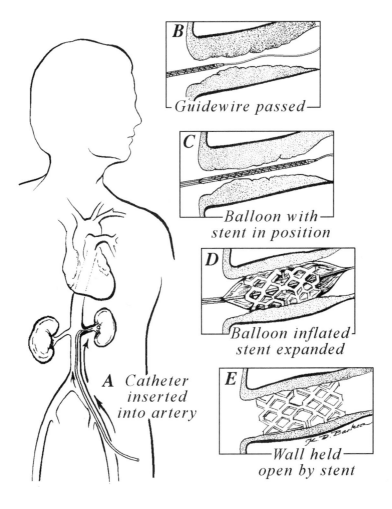

Figure 80 - This endovascular procedure is used for most cases of renal artery stenosis. The objectives of such surgery are to remove the obstruction, restore the blood flow to normal, decrease the elevated blood pressure, and preserve the function of the kidney.

Bypass Grafts to Renal Arteries

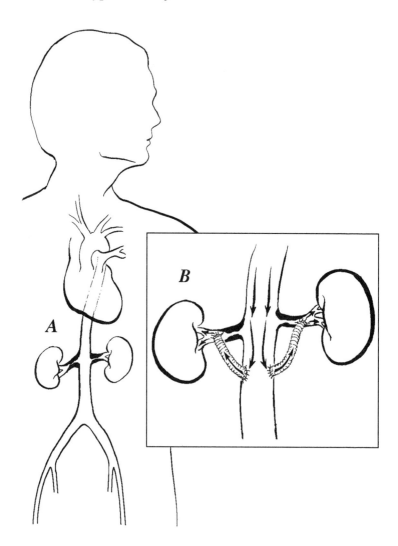

Figure 81 - (A) Bilateral stenosis of renal arteries. (B) Bypass grafts to renal arteries beyond the sites of obstruction carry red blood from the aorta to the kidneys, restoring flow, decreasing the elevated blood pressure, and preserving the function of the kidneys.

Surgery to Increase
the Blood Flow to the Legs

Obstruction of blood flow to the legs may occur from blockages of the arteries in the abdomen, at the groins, in the thighs, at the knees, and in the lower legs. These obstructions can occur at more than one site in the same patient and may be partial or complete. Both vascular and endovascular operations are important in the management of these problems.

The location and extent of the blockages determines which operation will be best for the patient. For obstructions of the abdominal aorta and/or the iliac arteries, vascular operations performed within the abdomen either to remove the thickened inner wall and clot or to implant synthetic grafts that bypass the blockages have proven to be reliable procedures to increase the blood supply to the legs.

When the iliac artery blood flow is good on one side and poor in the other, a synthetic graft can be placed to connect the leg arteries at the groin (common femorals), enabling the good side to supply red blood to the pelvis and both legs.

For high risk patients whose iliac flow is low on both sides, a graft can be placed from the artery of an arm at the shoulder to the main artery of the leg at the groin on the same side and joined there to a graft which connects to the main artery in the other groin. This enables the arm artery to supply red blood to the pelvis and both legs.

Today, endovascular operations are preferred to reopen the blocked channels of the aorta and/or iliac arteries. This is accomplished by dilating narrowed sites with balloons, dissolving clots with drugs, and placing stents when needed.

If the thigh artery becomes blocked gradually as it runs from the groin to the knee, nature can usually build a satisfactory "bypass" of its own by developing collateral vessels to carry blood around the obstruction and enable the person to still lead a reasonably active life.

But there are some individuals whose collateral circulation isn't adequate and, if the blockage is over two inches in length, placement of a bypass graft from the artery at the groin to the artery near the knee is the best way to restore circulation.

For shorter obstructions, endovascular operations employing balloons (often with stents) to open the arterial channel from the inside have become accepted practice today even though the frequency of recurrent blockage is much higher than that of bypass grafts made from the patient's veins.

If a surgeon implants an artificial graft to carry blood around an obstructed artery in the thigh of a patient who has sticky platelets that don't respond to aspirin or other medications, that graft will likely fill with clot after a few months and fail. For these patients, a superficial vein taken from the patient's leg or arm should be used as the graft, because the blood flowing through it will not clot unless the flow becomes very slow.

But if an individual's platelets aren't sticky or can be made to become that way by medications, that person's blood will likely be unable to clot off an artificial graft. In such patients, artificial grafts constructed of Dacron yarn, expanded teflon, or other acceptable artificial materials can be used to bypass the occluded artery in the thigh with a high expectation of long-term success. The advantage of using artificial grafts under these circumstances is that the patient's veins can be saved to bypass the arteries of the heart or lower legs, should this become necessary.

When the arteries below the knee are blocked in addition to those at the knee and in the thigh, the impairment of circulation to the foot is usually so marked that the patient is at high risk to lose the leg unless the circulation can be increased. In such circumstances, long-length grafts can often be placed from the big artery at the groin to a small artery near the ankle or even in the foot. By far the best graft for this demanding purpose is one of the patient's superficial veins, taken from a leg or an arm.

Endovascular operations are seldom applicable in the small vessels far below the knee, and, if attempted, are rarely successful. In fact, the closer to the foot a revascularization procedure has to be performed, the greater the necessity to use a healthy, living vein as the bypass graft. This is because the blood flowing through even the best of artificial grafts will clot long before it would in a natural vessel lined by healthy endothelial cells.

Sometimes procedures are required at two levels to adequately restore the blood flow to the lower extremities. Such combinations may involve two grafts -- for example, one graft placed from the big artery in the abdomen, the aorta, to the artery at the groin, the femoral, and another graft placed from there to the artery at the knee, the popliteal, bypassing obstructions in the abdomen and in the thigh. Endovascular and open vascular operations may also be combined -- for example, using a balloon angioplasty procedure to open a blocked common iliac artery in the abdomen and then using a graft from the artery at the groin to the artery at the knee to bypass a blocked thigh artery.

Aortobifemoral (Abdomen-to-Groin) Bypass

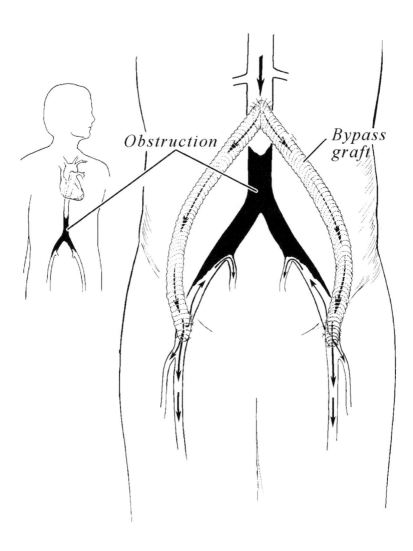

Figure 82 - Obstruction of the aorta and common iliac arteries blocks the flow of blood to the pelvis and legs. A bypass graft from the aorta above the blockage to the femoral arteries below carries a new supply of red blood to the pelvis and the legs.

Crossover Femorofemoral (Leg-to-Leg) Bypass

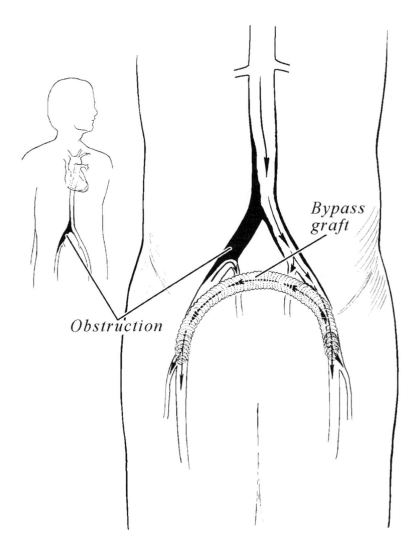

Figure 83 - In this instance, the right common iliac artery is closed, but the left is fully open. Placing a synthetic graft from the femoral artery in the groin on the open side to the femoral artery in the groin on the closed side enables the open side to supply red blood to the pelvis and both legs.

Axillofemoral (Arm-to-Leg) Bypass

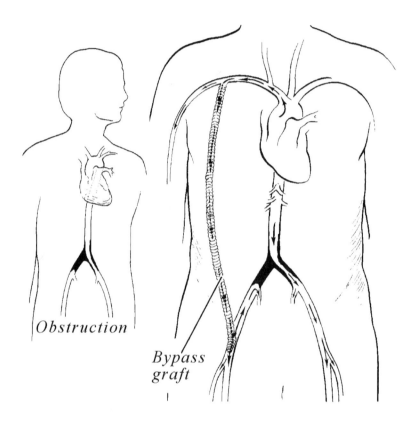

Obstruction

*Bypass
graft*

*Figure 84 - Threatening decrease of the blood supply to the right
leg due to complete occlusion of the right common iliac arteries in
an elderly, fragile patient presents a problem when the blood
supply to the left leg is too low to also supply the right leg through
a leg-to-leg graft at the groin. Under these circumstances,
diverting red blood to the femoral artery at the right groin from the
axillary artery going to the right arm through a graft called an
"axillofemoral bypass" is an effective operation that the elderly
patient can tolerate. The right leg gains much needed blood supply,
and the supply of the right arm is not impaired.*

Combined Axillofemoral (Arm-to-Leg) and Crossover Femorofemoral (Leg-to-Leg) Bypass

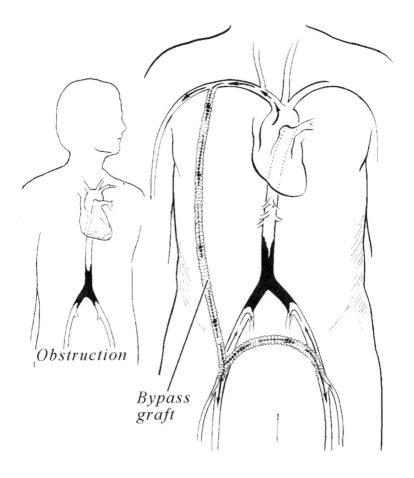

Obstruction

Bypass
graft

Figure 85 - For frail patients who are in need of increased circulation to the lower half of the body but can't have a more major vascular or endovascular operation, the combination of an arm-to-leg graft on one side with a leg-to-leg graft to the opposite side is an effective operation that relieves pain, avoids ulcers, and enables these fragile patients to walk within their limited general capacity. This procedure brings red blood to the pelvis and both legs.

Balloon Angioplasty with Primary Stent Placement for Narrowed Common Iliac Artery

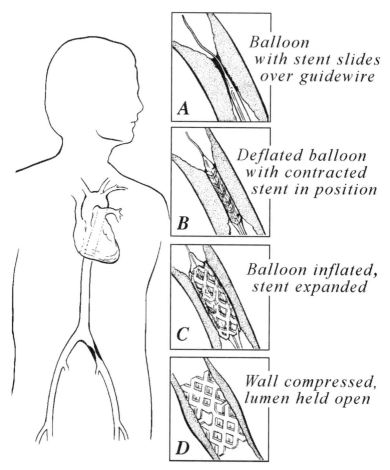

Balloon with stent slides over guidewire

A

Deflated balloon with contracted stent in position

B

Balloon inflated, stent expanded

C

Wall compressed, lumen held open

D

Figure 86 - Endovascular surgery using an inflatable balloon-tipped catheter to dilate areas of narrowing in the common iliac arteries is now frequently followed by stent placement to compact the wall and expand the lumen. This procedure has largely replaced open vascular surgery (removal of the inner wall or placement of a bypass graft) for treatment of this lesion. Shown here is use of the balloon technique with primary stent placement to increase the flow of red blood to the pelvis and leg.

Endarterectomy of the Arteries at the Groin

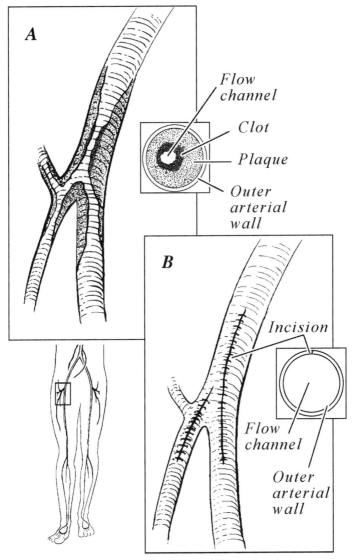

Figure 87 - Endarterectomy (Fig. 61, p. 196) of the blocked arteries at the groin and upper thigh increases the flow of red blood to the thigh and lower leg.

Nature's "Operation" for Gradual Occlusion of the Thigh Artery

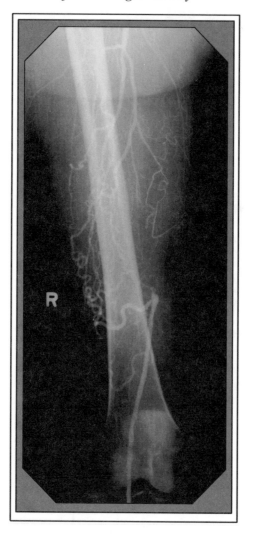

Figure 88 - As this patient's thigh artery became gradually blocked, such extensive collateral circulation developed that it could supply enough red blood to the leg to support nearly full activity. Exciting new developments with gene therapy may enable nature to build even bigger vessels faster, even in the heart.

Balloon Angioplasty with Primary Stent Placement for Narrowed Short Segment of the Lower Superficial Femoral (Thigh) Artery

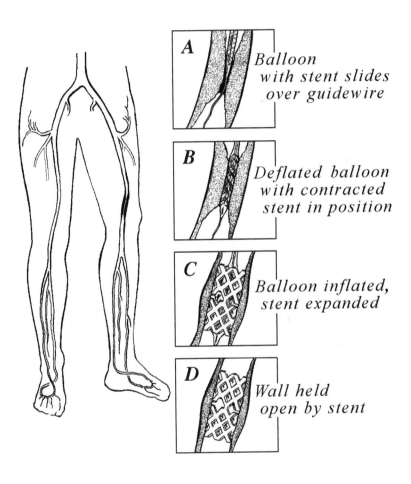

A Balloon with stent slides over guidewire

B Deflated balloon with contracted stent in position

C Balloon inflated, stent expanded

D Wall held open by stent

Figure 89 - Shown here is the use of the balloon technique with primary stent placement to open a short, narrowed segment of the main artery in the lower thigh.

Groin-to-Above-Knee (Femoropopliteal) Bypass Using a Synthetic Graft for Long Segment Blockage of the Superficial Femoral (Thigh) Artery

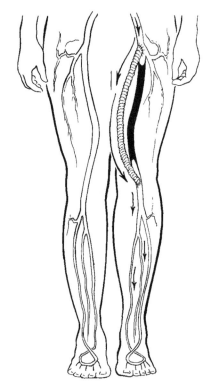

Figure 90 - Blockage of the superficial femoral artery in the thigh of a patient whose sticky platelets were made non-sticky by one regular aspirin a day. A bypass graft placed from the artery at the groin to the artery above the knee delivers needed red blood to the lower leg. A synthetic graft could be safely used in this patient because the patient's sticky platelets became much less sticky with aspirin. If the platelets hadn't changed, a vein graft would have been used instead. This patient will continue to take one aspirin each day indefinitely to keep the platelets from becoming sticky.

Groin-to-Below-Knee (Femoropopliteal) Bypass Using a Vein Graft for Long Segment Blockage of the Superficial Femoral (Thigh) and Upper Popliteal (Knee) Arteries

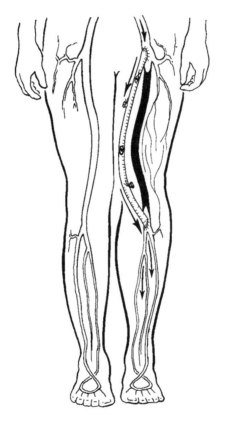

Figure 91 - Blockage of the superficial femoral and upper popliteal arteries severely impairs the supply of red blood to the lower leg. The saphenous vein from this leg is placed as a graft from the artery at the groin to the artery below the knee. This graft conveys the needed red blood to the lower leg and is resistant to clot formation because of the healthy endothelial cells that cover its flow surface.

Groin-to-Lower-Leg (Femorotibial) Bypass Using a Long Vein Graft

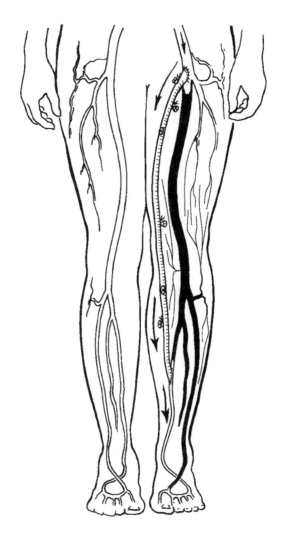

Figure 92 - Obstruction of the main leg arteries all the way to the foot except for one vessel in the lower leg. A long vein graft from the big artery at the groin to this open vessel provides an adequate supply of red blood to save the extremity and restore function.

Groin-to-Foot (Femoropedal) Bypass Using a Very Long Vein Graft

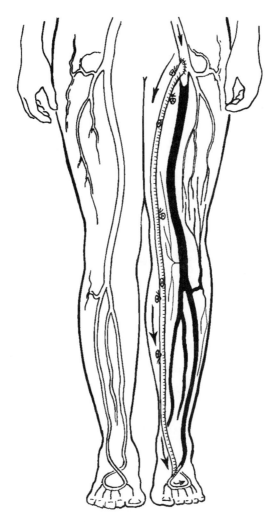

Figure 93 - Obstruction of the main arteries all the way to the foot critically impairs the blood supply to the lower leg and foot. Even so, in most cases, a very long vein graft from the big artery at the groin to a small artery in the foot provides an adequate supply of red blood to save the extremity and restore function.

Surgery for Aortic Aneurysms

The reason for removing an aortic aneurysm is to prevent fatal hemorrhage from rupture. In the most common technique, a synthetic graft is placed inside the aneurysm and sewn to the arterial wall above and below the ballooned-out segment. The remaining outer wall of the aneurysm is trimmed and then sutured to itself to form a tight tissue covering around the graft.

Graft for Thoracic Aneurysm

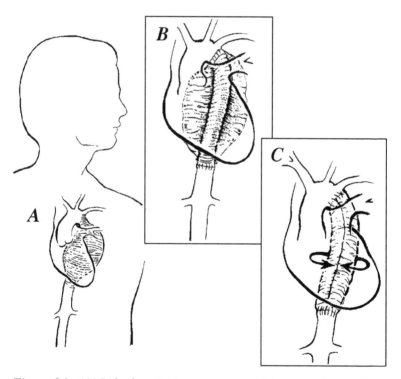

Figure 94 - (A) Life-threatening aneurysm of the aorta in the chest. (B) Aneurysm repaired by a Dacron graft placed inside the weakened and ballooned-out wall. (C) Outer wall of aneurysm sutured around graft.

Graft for Abdominal Aneurysm

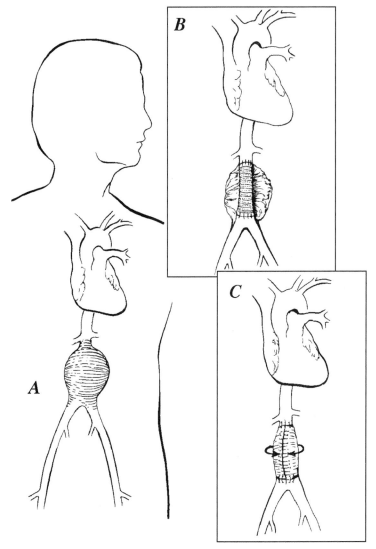

Figure 95 - (A) Life-threatening aneurysm of the aorta in the abdomen. (B) Aneurysm repaired by a Dacron graft placed inside the weakened and ballooned-out wall, preserving the aortic bifurcation. (C) Outer wall of aneurysm sutured around graft.

Section VI:

Related Heart Topics

The Pacemaking and Conducting
  Systems of the Heart 243-245

Artificial Pacemakers for the Heart 246-249

Cardiopulmonary Resuscitation (CPR)..............................250-252

The Automatic Internal Cardiac Defibrillator 253-255

Heart Transplantation 256-258

The Pacemaking and Conducting Systems of the Heart

The pacing system of the heart is made up of special cells that build up an electric charge -- discharge it over the conducting system -- build up another charge -- discharge it -- and continue to do this indefinitely. The cells that fire fastest set the rate of the heartbeat.

The electrical impulses that originate from the pacemaking cells spread over the special pathways of the conducting system to reach the muscle cells of the heart and cause them to contract in a coordinated manner that enables the right ventricle to pump the blue blood to the lungs and the left ventricle to pump the red blood to the rest of the body.

The pacing cells that fire fastest are in a structure called the *sinus node*, which is located in the top portion of the front wall of the right atrium where the superior vena cava enters to return the blue blood from the upper part of the body. With sedentary activity these cells build up and discharge an electrical impulse about 80 times a minute to drive the heart. During exercise these cells discharge at a faster rate; during sleep they discharge at a somewhat slower rate.

If the sinus node cells lose their pacing ability, the next cells further along in the pacing system take over at their slower rate. Then, if these cells lose their pacing ability, the next cells down the line take over, etc., the pulse rate becoming progressively slower as this happens.

The Pacemaking and Conducting Systems of the Heart

Sinus node

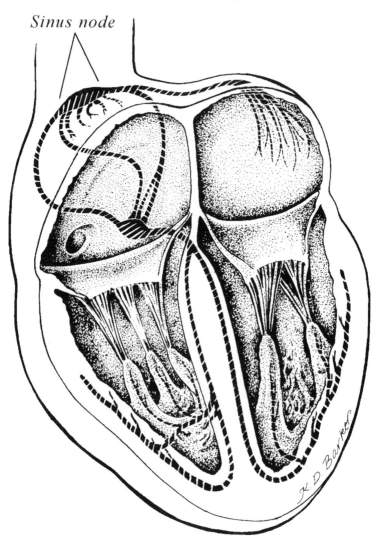

Figure 96 - Normally, the electrical impulses that cause the heart to contract arise in the sinus node and spread from there in an orderly sequence to cause the atria to beat first and then the ventricles.

Sometimes when the sinus node cells lose their ability to pace the heart, the beat becomes so slow that the decreased circulation causes the patient to become weak and dizzy. The heart may even stop. If it stops for more than 10 seconds, the patient will lose consciousness because when the heart is stopped the brain receives no oxygen.

Fortunately, when this happens, the cells of the sinus node or of some other site further down the pacing system will generally start firing within 15 to 20 seconds, restoring the heart beat and the circulation. With the return of circulation, the brain receives oxygen and glucose and quickly regains its function. Within seconds the patient awakens with no recollection of having been unconscious.

When the heart stops, there is always danger it may not start again or that it may start too late. If the heart should stop for four or more minutes, the lack of oxygen during the arrest period would irreparably damage the brain cells.

Malfunction of the pacing and conduction system of the heart affects millions of people worldwide. Prior to the development of the early pacemakers in the 1950's, these difficult and often deadly problems could only be treated by medicines that were usually ineffective.

Artificial Pacemakers
for the Heart

Artificial pacemakers have been developed to treat patients who can't function normally because their heart rates are too slow or who are in danger of death from their hearts stopping. Pacemakers consist of two main components: a miniaturized battery (pulse generator) with electronic sensing and firing mechanisms packaged in a metal container and one or two electrodes with long leads. Each electrode with its attached lead is inserted into a vein and advanced into the right side of the heart where it attaches to the inner wall. The other end of the lead is inserted into the connecting port of the pulse generator.

After these connections are completed, the pulse generator is placed beneath the fatty layer of the anterior chest wall a short way below the collarbone. The attachment of the lead or leads to the heart on one end and to the pulse generator on the other enables this unit to monitor the electrical activity of the heart and when necessary, to serve as its pacemaker. This function is painless to the patient who is unaware when the artificial pacemaker is firing.

When the pacemaking cells discharge an impulse and cause the muscle cells to contract, electric currents are generated. The electrocardiogram (ECG) is a record of these electrical events. The electrode(s) attached to the inner surface of the heart transmit a continuous ECG back over the lead(s) to the sensing mechanism in the pulse generator. This mechanism monitors the heart's action, and if the preset level for firing is reached the generator discharges electric impulses that travel rapidly over the lead(s) to the electrode(s) from where these impulses spread to the muscle cells throughout the heart and stimulate them to contract.

Artificial Ventricular Pacemaker for the Heart

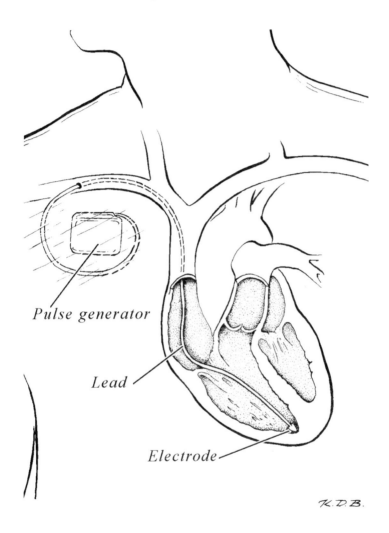

Pulse generator

Lead

Electrode

K.D.B.

Figure 97 - A single electrode is positioned in the right ventricle where it monitors the electrical activity of the heart, and if the heart rate falls below the pacemaker's setting the pulse generator fires at its preset rate and stimulates the ventricles to contract.

These electronic units can be programmed to keep the heartbeat from dropping below any rate that is selected. For example, if the activation rate of the pacer is set at 70, and the patient's heart rate drops below 70, the pacer senses this immediately and begins firing at its preset rate of 70 times a minute. Each time the pacer fires the heart contracts in response to the electrical impulse and pumps blood to the lungs and body. The pacer is now the heart's pacemaker. When the patient's natural heart rate again becomes faster than that of the pacer, the pacer returns to its "sensing" only mode and waits -- ever ready to be called into action.

Today, there are many sophisticated pacemakers that function so superbly that they are able to effectively treat nearly all of the pacing problems that patients experience. Many modern pacemakers have two leads, one that is positioned in the right atrium and one in the right ventricle. With these leads, the pacer is able to monitor the electrical activity of both the atria and the ventricles and pace them to function in a normal, integrated manner when called on to do so.

Some pacemakers are activity-responsive and fire faster when the patient exercises and slower when the patient rests.

Implanting a pacemaker is usually an easy procedure done under local anesthesia. These amazing devices have now been implanted in millions of patients worldwide. Last year approximately 120,000 pacemakers were implanted in the United States alone. Most of these units are warranted by the manufacturers for five years, but today many are expected to last 10 or more years before the pulse generator will need to be changed. Changing the generator is a simple operation done with local anesthesia in outpatient surgery.

Artificial Combined Atrial and Ventricular Pacemakers for the Heart

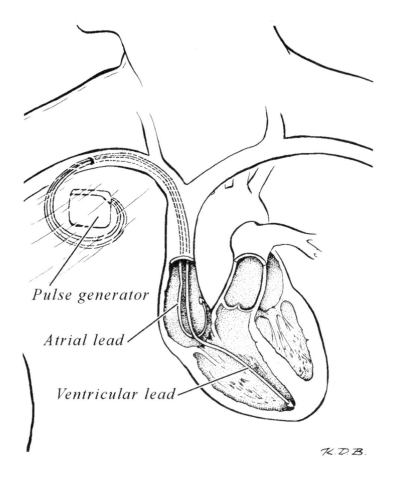

Pulse generator

Atrial lead

Ventricular lead

K. D. B.

Figure 98 - This pacemaker with two electrodes, one positioned in the right atrium and the other in the right ventricle, stimulates the atria to contract first and then the ventricles in a normal time sequence. The output of the heart with this type of pacemaker is significantly higher than with pacemakers that pace only the ventricles.

Cardiopulmonary Resuscitation (CPR)

When the heart stops, cardiopulmonary resuscitation (CPR) is the emergency procedure employed to get the circulation going again before the most sensitive organ, the brain, is damaged by lack of oxygen. Circulatory stoppage for as short a time as four minutes will cause severe brain damage. For people whose hearts stop, their survival depends largely on how quickly they are found and what the first person who finds them does.

The heart may stop in one of two ways. It may suddenly cease beating and lie still, showing no motion. This type of stoppage is called *cardiac arrest.* More commonly, when the heart stops beating, it develops a wiggling type of uncoordinated motion that is unable to pump blood. This type of stoppage is called *ventricular fibrillation.*

To be successful, CPR must get oxygen into and carbon dioxide out of the blood and then pump this life-giving fluid to the tissues where it sustains them until the heart regains its beat and the patient is breathing again in an adequate manner. In the usual case of heart stoppage that occurs outside the hospital, the person performing CPR alternately ventilates the lungs by mouth-to-mouth respiration and then pumps this refreshed blood (replenished with oxygen and depleted of carbon dioxide) to the tissues by pushing the lower portion of the breastbone (sternum) inward to compress the heart.

If one day you should hear a thud in the adjacent room and on investigation find that someone, perhaps your husband or wife, has collapsed, is unconscious, isn't breathing, and has no pulse, grab the phone and call 911. Ask them to come

Cardiopulmonary Resuscitation (CPR)

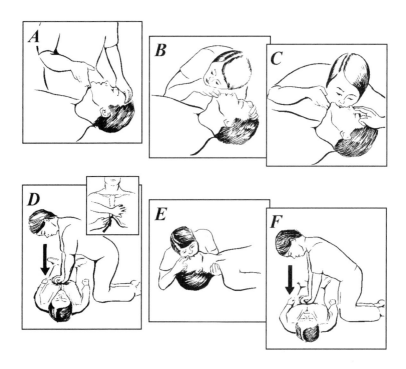

Figure 99 - (A) After giving a strong thump to the chest over the heart, tilt the patient's chin up and rotate the head back to hold the airway open. (B & C) If the patient still isn't breathing and has no pulse, pinch the nose shut and give two deep mouth-to-mouth breaths (1 to 2 seconds per breath) while holding the airway open. (D) Then compress the lower sternum sharply inward 15 times at a rate of about one compression every 2/3 of a second. (E & F) Continue this "breathe and compress" sequence until the heart is beating and the patient is breathing or until help arrives to relieve you. CPR can be continued for an hour or more with complete recovery.

immediately to your address. *It's valuable to **practice** this **call**, because in an emergency any of us can mentally block and forget 911, our phone number, and even our address. Try it now! When it's for real, **seconds count.***

Then quickly turn the patient on his/her back, and lift the chin up with one hand while rotating the forehead back with your other hand to extend the neck. This moves the lower jaw forward and lifts the tongue and epiglottis away from the back of the throat to open the airway. Now follow the "breathe and compress" sequence given in Fig. 99.

If two people are available to resuscitate the patient, one tends to the lungs and the other to the heart. In this situation, the person tending to the breathing gives one big breath over about two seconds and then waits while the person tending to the heart gives five sternal compressions at a rate of about one every 2/3 second. The two-person team continues this 5:1 cycle until professional help arrives or the patient's heartbeat and breathing have returned.

The arrested heart will often begin to beat after starting CPR, but this doesn't happen with heart stoppage due to ventricular fibrillation. Electric shock is required to stop fibrillation, but this must await the arrival of the emergency medical technician team in response to your 911 call. Generally, they will arrive within minutes to take over CPR from you. If the heart is fibrillating, the team will get the heart in the best possible condition and then shock it with a *defibrillator* to stop the fibrillation.

After the heart is beating again, the patient is taken to an appropriate hospital for intensive care and later investigation to determine what caused the heart to stop and what can be done to prevent it from stopping again.

The Automatic Internal Cardiac Defibrillator (AICD)

An automatic internal cardiac defibrillator (AICD) is like a pacemaker, only its battery is bigger and more powerful, and its electronic sensing and firing mechanisms are programmed to detect and treat ventricular fibrillation rather than a slow heart rate.

Several years ago, two electrodes were required to defibrillate the heart, and they were so big that the chest had to be opened to place them on the outside of the heart. Today only one electrode is needed, and this electrode has been made sufficiently small that it can be inserted into a vein -- like the lead of a pacemaker -- and advanced into the chambers of the right side of the heart. The other end of this special lead is inserted into the connecting port of the pulse generator, and this unit is then placed beneath the fatty layer of the anterior chest wall a short distance below the collarbone in a similar position to that employed for the smaller pulse generator of a pacemaker.

Automatic internal cardiac defibrillators have now been implanted in hundreds of thousands of patients around the world who are at high risk of sudden death from their hearts developing ventricular fibrillation. Because the ventricles are the main pumping chambers of the heart, when they arrest or fibrillate, the circulation stops.

Typically, a patient with an implanted defibrillator whose heart arrests or fibrillates begins to feel faint within a few seconds of the stoppage and would soon fall to the floor unconscious if it were not for activation of the defibrillator electrode connected to the heart. The sensing mechanism of the unit diagnoses what is wrong and quickly treats it.

The Automatic Internal Cardiac Defibrillator (AICD)

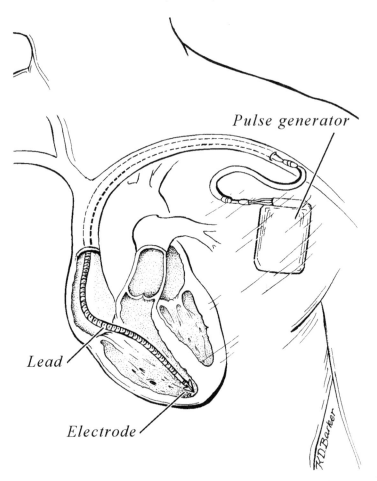

Figure 100 - The automatic internal cardiac defibrillator (AICD) monitors the electrical activity of the heart, and if ventricular fibrillation occurs, the generator discharges a strong electrical impulse that shocks the heart and stops the fibrillation. Usually the heart quickly regains its beat, but if it does not, the generator paces the ventricles like a pacemaker.

If the heart has arrested, the pulse generator of the AICD unit discharges an appropriate impulse that paces the heart like a conventional pacemaker. If the sensing mechanism detects that the ventricles are fibrillating, the pulse generator discharges a stronger impulse that stops the fibrillation.

After a few seconds, the still heart usually starts to beat. But if it does not, the sensing mechanism recognizes this and activates the pacing cycle.

With the return of the heart beat, the circulation begins to deliver oxygen and glucose to the brain. As this happens, the patient's sense of faintness disappears. When the heart is beating on its own at an adequate rate, the AICD unit returns to its "sensing only" mode.

There is no question that further major technologic advances may be expected in this dynamic field. Recent developments include pacemaker-AICD combinations and implantable defibrillators for atrial fibrillation.

Heart Transplantation

Heart transplantation has become an excellent treatment for patients whose hearts are worn out and can't be repaired. But the main factor limiting greater use of this operation is the small number of donor hearts that are available. In the United States there are only about 2,500 donor hearts that are suitable for transplantation which become available each year. The need is much greater. Tens of thousands die for lack of a donor heart.

The best donor hearts come from young accident victims with healthy hearts whose brain function has been destroyed by massive head injuries. If the family consents to their loved one's organs being used for the benefit of others, the donor's body is kept alive on a respirator for a few days while transplant matches are established with potential heart, lung, liver, kidney, and pancreas recipients who are usually within 500 miles of the donor's location.

We shall now comment specifically about transplantation of the human heart.

When all the arrangements for the heart transplant have been made, the procurement team from the recipient's center flies to the donor's city and removes the donor's beating heart. The heart is rinsed free of blood, cooled to 4°C, and kept at that temperature while the team flies back to deliver the cold, pale, limp heart to the implant team in the operating room where the recipient is ready to be placed on bypass using the heart-lung machine.

It's now "**Go!**" The surgical team moves rapidly. Bypass is begun. The patient's old, sick heart is removed and the donor's new healthy one is sutured in its place.

Heart Transplantation

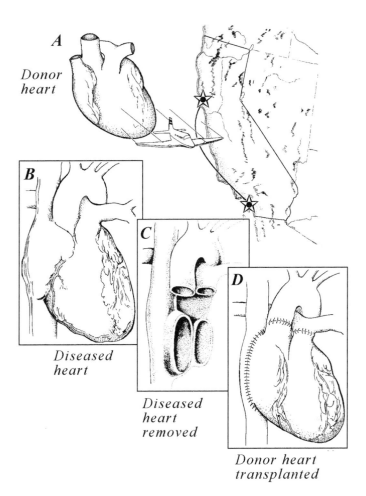

A

Donor
heart

B

Diseased
heart

C

Diseased
heart
removed

D

Donor heart
transplanted

Figure 101 - In this case, the procurement team from Los Angeles flies to San Francisco and removes the heart from a brain-dead donor. This team flies back to Los Angeles and delivers the heart to the implant team waiting in the operating room. The surgical team then proceeds rapidly to place the patient on heart-lung bypass, remove the recipient's worn-out heart, and implant the donor's healthy heart in its place.

With the new heart sutured in position, the decisive moment has now arrived . . . the clamp is removed from the patient's aorta. The unspoken question, "Will the heart beat?" is foremost in everyone's mind as the warm, red blood flows into the coronary arteries and begins to return color, warmth, and function to the transplanted heart.

As the blood surges through the coronaries, the heart becomes pink and often without an electric shock suddenly starts to beat and restores the pulse of life.

As this happens, all in the operating room breathe a sign of relief and thank God for answering their silent prayers.

As the heart gains strength, the surgeon directs the perfusionist running the heart-lung machine to progressively transfer the pumping of blood to the new heart. When the heart is doing all the work, the patient, now completely dependent on the transplant, begins a new life with the donor's gift at the center of his or her physical being.

After the wound bleeding has been stopped, the surgical team closes the chest. Then, when the anesthesiologist is satisfied with the patient's condition, the patient is taken to the cardiac intensive care unit. Within a short time, the patient awakens and the miracle of life continues.

Today, about 80% of the patients who received a heart transplant five years ago are doing well. Fifteen years ago, such results were but a dream. The research of yesterday made this advance possible by discovering safer and more effective drugs to prevent the patient's immune system from rejecting the donor's heart. Research yet to be done will make tomorrow's results even better.

Section VII:

Spiritual Reflections

It is fitting to conclude this book about the physical structure of our intricate human bodies by pausing to reflect on the spiritual aspects of our eternal lives. We are more than mere matter; we are body and soul, created by God for all eternity. It is appropriate, therefore, that we each seek inspiration for maintaining the health of our mortal bodies by also considering the health of our immortal souls.

We suggest that as strength and vigor are hallmarks of robust physical health, peace and joy are indications of vibrant spiritual well-being. There is now no doubt that such a spiritual state has a positive influence on our physical condition. God gives this joyful state to us when we serve those who need us out of our open hearts in a spirit of love.

Although most of us feel quite comfortable talking and thinking about the importance of taking good care of our physical bodies, it is rare that we stop to assess our spiritual status. As a result of failing to do this, we tend to merely exist rather than truly live. Though there is real mental work in pausing to face this vital issue, the reward is worth the effort. The appreciation of our life's purpose, value, and spiritual destiny is at stake. And further, our **happiness**

. . . that priceless peace of mind, serenity of soul, and
exhilaration of spirit . . .

depends on what we do in response to this appreciation.

A powerful attraction of all the great religions is the simplicity of the means they advocate for obtaining happiness . . . loving one's neighbor as oneself. Love in this context may, perhaps, best be defined as the giving of oneself for the benefit of another.

Christ set the example of love for humankind by becoming one of us in a stable at Bethlehem and in dying for us on a cross atop Calvary. He gave us clear direction when He said, "Whatsoever you do unto the least of these, you do unto Me." The world's other great religions -- including Judaism, Hinduism, Buddhism, and Islam -- all convey similar messages. They teach in different yet similar ways that a life barren of love is devoid of real meaning and true happiness.

In this context, we should see ourselves broadly as members of one worldwide human family, rather than isolated, for example, as Christians, Jews, or Buddhists; or as Americans, Russians, or Chinese. Each of us, in love with our God -- no matter what religious tradition we follow -- can become an increasingly effective instrument of God's ministry to all people by serving those in need out of love. This call to serve God by serving humanity is ever before us. We will all find purpose, worth, and happiness in our lives if we do this.

The holy scriptures of all the major religions come together in their teaching that each of us is unique in our own way, and that there is a divine purpose for every human life. And that divine purpose is to love and serve God by serving humanity out of love. God waits within our soul for us to find and follow Him on this path of human service. When we do, God rewards us with that pristine state of consciousness in which we experience peace, joy, and happiness.

Through the perspective of medicine, as in no other field of human endeavor, our lives are clearly seen to be time-limited. And in medicine, one is awed by the "Something Greater Than Ourselves" that is responsible for our human existence and everything around us.

In writing this book and preparing its illustrations, we have felt the wonder of the spiritual essence that is in all of us. In reading this book, we hope that you have felt it, too.

Our progress through life and the degree of happiness we derive from this journey to eternity and what we'll find when we get there will be largely determined by the road we travel in this life. Will it be the way of hatred, envy, greed, and anger or the less traveled route of love, joy, peace, and compassion? The choice is ours.

To attain the priceless treasures of spiritual peace and joy, we must first see God in the soul of every human being, including ourselves. Only when this has become reality to us will we be able to follow the request of the Holy Spirit to tend His flock. To do this is the ultimate challenge and true adventure of our lives.

Together, let us pray that God will guide and bless us through all the days of the rest of our lives so that we will understand who we are, appreciate our purpose, value our true worth, and serve God out of our open hearts by helping those in need. Mother Teresa said it so beautifully, "It's not how much we do, but how much love we put in what we do that counts with God."

To conclude this section, let us take the immortal words of St. Francis of Assisi into our hearts as we continue our earthly journeys to eternity:

Prayer of St. Francis

Lord, make me an instrument
of your peace.

Where there is hatred,
let me sow love;
Where there is injury, pardon;
Where there is doubt, faith;
Where there is despair, hope;
Where there is darkness, light;
And where there is sadness, joy.

O Divine Master, grant that I may not
so much seek to be consoled as to console;
to be understood as to understand;
to be loved as to love.

For it is in giving that we receive,
it is in pardoning that we are pardoned,
and it is in dying
that we are born to eternal life.

Section VIII:
Glossary

Aneurysm
An arterial segment that has ballooned (bulged) out because its wall has become weak due to disease or injury. The bulging occurs because the pressure of the blood within the flow channel stretches the weakened wall. Aneurysms are most common in the big artery in the abdomen, the aorta. The wall of an aortic aneurysm will usually continue to stretch until the pressure of the blood within it eventually ruptures the wall and causes massive hemorrhage.

Angina Pectoris
Pain felt in the left anterior chest wall due to an insufficient supply of oxygenated (red) blood to the heart muscle.

Anticoagulants
Drugs which delay clotting of the blood (coagulation). When given in cases where a blood vessel is plugged up by a clot, anticoagulants act to prevent new clots from forming and existing clots from enlarging, but they don't dissolve clots.

Aorta
The biggest artery in the body. It arises from the outlet of the left side of the heart and arches up above it like the handle of a cane that is directed to the back and left side of the chest near the midline. The aorta then passes downward through the back of the chest and abdomen, coming to lie in front of the spine in the lower portion. The aorta gives off many branches which carry blood to all parts of the body. At the level of the umbilicus, the aorta divides into the right and left common iliac arteries which descend to supply their side of the pelvis and the leg below.

Aortogram
An x-ray examination of the aorta made after injecting dye into the blood that shows the channel of this large vessel and its branches.

Arrhythmia
Any variation from the normal rhythm of the heartbeat.

Arteries
The vessels that carry blood away from the heart. The pulmonary arteries convey the deoxygenated (blue) blood pumped out by the right ventricle to the lungs where it takes up oxygen, gives off carbon dioxide, and becomes red. The systemic arteries convey the oxygenated (red) blood pumped out by the left ventricle to the cells of the body where it gives off oxygen, takes up carbon dioxide, and becomes blue. The arterial wall has three layers (intima-- inner portion, media -- middle portion, and adventitia -- outer portion).

Atherosclerosis (Hardening of the Arteries)
A disease of epidemic proportions in industrialized, developed countries where it causes more deaths than all types of cancer, accidents, and infections combined. It is due in large measure to smoking; eating too much saturated fat, *trans* fatty acids, sugar, and low-fiber complex carbohydrates; taking in too many calories; leading a sedentary life; gaining excess weight (fat); and letting stress control and distort our lives.

In most patients, this disease causes the inner portion of the arterial wall to become thick, inelastic, and hardened due to plaques formed by infiltration of LDL cholesterol, fat, and variable amounts of calcium from the blood. Plaques with lots of calcification are hard and those with little are soft. Many soft plaques develop a central collection (core) of thick, slimy, fatty fluid that is covered over by a thin cap of fibrous tissue. If the cap ruptures, the deadly, syrupy liquid in the core oozes into the flow channel where it can cause the blood to clot. This is the most common cause of heart attacks.

Atherosclerosis often makes the arterial flow surface lose its delicate lining of endothelial cells as the inner wall becomes rough, irregular, and ulcerated. If the blood flow slows or becomes turbulent, the diseased flow surface may cause clots to form which block the channel and stop the flow of blood. Whether by this process or by rupture of a soft plaque with a lipid core, the flow channel can become blocked by clot and cause heart attacks, strokes, high blood pressure, impaired walking, and amputations.

In a lesser number of patients, the atherosclerotic process weakens the arterial wall so much, most commonly of the aorta in the abdomen, that the blood pressure forces the wall to bulge out and form enlargements called aneurysms, which may rupture and cause fatal hemorrhage.

There is a current suspicion, as yet insufficiently proven, that the bacterium, *Chlamydia pneumoniae,* as well as some viruses, may infect the arterial wall and be part of the "hardened" artery problem. The question of which comes first, like the chicken or the egg, will be the subject of much future research.

Blood Pressure -- Arterial (systemic)
The force that the flowing blood exerts against the arterial wall. Two pressures are measured:

The *systolic pressure.* This is the highest pressure that occurs in the arteries when the heart contracts and pumps the red blood out into the aorta.

The *diastolic pressure.* This is the lowest pressure that occurs in the arteries while the heart is filling in preparation for its next beat.

Capillaries

The tiniest blood vessels. Capillary networks connect the smallest arteries to the smallest veins. The capillaries wind between and around the cells to bring them what they need and remove what they don't need. No cell can be further away from its feeding capillary than the width of the finest hair.

Capillary walls are composed of a single layer of endothelial cells through which oxygen, water, nutrients, and other chemicals diffuse from the blood into the cells throughout the body, while carbon dioxide and other waste products diffuse from the cells into the blood.

Carbohydrates (plant foods -- see Fiber, pages 274-275)

Organic compounds constructed of carbon, hydrogen, and oxygen, usually in a ratio of 1:2:1. Most of these compounds are polysaccharides which are called complex carbohydrates. They are broken down in the body by the digestive enzymes into the monosaccharide, glucose($C_6H_{12}O_6$), which is absorbed into the blood and transported to the cells where it is used to produce energy. The brain cells and the cells of the retina can only use glucose for energy; other cells can also use fatty acids.

Excess glucose in plants and animals is stored in the same form $(C_6H_{10}O_5)x$, called starch in plants and glycogen in animals. *Insulin,* a hormone secreted by the pancreas, enables the cells to use glucose for energy and converts the excess glucose into glycogen, which is stored 1/3 in the liver and 2/3 in muscles. A bit less than a pound of glycogen can be stored in the entire body. Above this level, glucose is rapidly converted into saturated fat and stored in the fat cells of the adipose tissue throughout the body. When extra energy is needed, *glucagon,* another hormone secreted by the pancreas, converts glycogen back into glucose. Insulin enables the cells to use this glucose for the energy they need.

Carbon Dioxide (CO_2)
This compound is formed in the cells when oxygen combines with carbon and releases energy. Carbon dioxide passes from the cells into the venous blood which carries it to the lungs. In the lungs the carbon dioxide diffuses into the tiny air sacs (the alveoli) where it is exhaled into the outside air.

Cardiac Arrest and
Ventricular Fibrillation
Cardiac arrest means that the heart suddenly stops beating and remains still. Ventricular fibrillation also means that the heart suddenly stops beating, but it doesn't lie still. Instead, the fibrillating heart at first wiggles vigorously, like a mass of angry angle worms. Then, as the oxygen and nutrient supplies are quickly exhausted, it moves less and less until after a few minutes the heart stops completely and lies motionless in a dilated, flaccid state.

In both conditions, no blood is pumped, and the blood pressure drops abruptly to zero. Unless the circulation can be restored within four minutes, the brain cells will be irreparably damaged by lack of oxygen. CPR -- Cardiopulmonary Resuscitation -- must be started before this happens. The fibrillating heart must usually be shocked into standstill with an electric current from an apparatus called a defibrillator before it can start beating again. With continued CPR, both the arrested heart and the defibrillated heart will usually start beating on their own.

Cardiologist
A doctor who specializes in the diagnosis and treatment of heart disease. Formerly cardiologists used only measures such as diet, drugs, exercise and rest to treat patients. Today many

cardiologists also pass catheters -- some with special devices attached to their distal ends (inflatable balloons, cutting instruments, rotating burrs, and ultrasound probes) -- into the coronary arteries and chambers of the heart both for the diagnosis and treatment of disease. In addition, cardiologists often pass leads with electronic components into the right side of the heart for pacemaking and defibrillation purposes.

Cardiopulmonary Resuscitation (CPR)
An emergency measure to maintain life when the heart stops. CPR consists of forcing air into the lungs by mouth-to-mouth respiration (or with a breathing bag if one is available) in a sequence alternating with pushing the lower part of the sternum inward against the front of the heart to restore the circulation. This "breathe and compress" sequence propels the blue blood returning from the body on through the right side of the heart into the lungs where it gains oxygen and loses carbon dioxide. CPR propels this blood, now red, on through the pulmonary veins into the left side of the heart and then on to all the cells of the body.

Cerebral Vascular Accident (CVA) (also known as **Stroke)**
This condition is more commonly referred to as a stroke or brain attack. Stroke patients show loss of brain function, such as the inability to move one side of the body, feel, speak, see, comprehend, and many other neurological deficits. Strokes are caused by blockage of the supply of red blood to some part of the brain. This obstruction is generally caused by one of the following three conditions:
1. an *embolus* -- a fragment of a clot, platelet clump, atherosclerotic plaque, or other material which breaks loose from the wall of the heart or artery and is carried by the blood to the brain where it blocks an artery.
2. a blood *clot* (thrombus) forming in an artery of the brain.
3. a brain *hemorrhage.*

Cholesterol

A fat-like substance used by the body in producing the retaining walls of all cells and in making the male and female sex hormones and the hormones secreted by the outer part (the cortex) of the adrenal gland in humans and animals.

Cholesterol is transported in the blood in one of two forms, high density lipoprotein cholesterol (HDL) and low density lipoprotein cholesterol (LDL). High concentrations of LDL, low concentrations of HDL, and high levels of triglycerides all predispose to the development of atherosclerosis. HDL cholesterol protects against the development of atherosclerosis by transporting LDL cholesterol out of the inner portion of the arterial wall and out of the lipid core of soft plaques to the liver which excretes it in the bile.

The conversion of saturated fat and *trans* fatty acids by the liver into LDL cholesterol is the main source of this chemical in our body. In addition, if we take in more calories than we use, our liver converts the excess (glucose and protein) into saturated fat. Some of this fat is converted into LDL cholesterol which, if the level rises above 100-120mg/dL, may infiltrate the inner wall of our arteries. This is the reason why it is so important to keep our weight under control and not allow the calories from saturated fat and *trans* fatty acids in our diet to exceed 10% of the total calories we consume in a day. Calorie wise, a little fat goes a long way. LDL cholesterol isn't a poison. It's bad only if it gets too high. It's a little like water. We can die of dehydration if we don't have enough, but we can drown in it if we have too much. We need the right amount.

Collateral Circulation

This is the blood that flows into the small branches that arise above a blockage and connect with the small vessels that originate below it. The blood flows through these vessels into the main artery below the blockage, or makes other connections, and from there supplies tissues downstream, to whatever extent possible. These connecting vessels are called *collateral vessels* and the blood that flows through them is called *collateral circulation.*

Common Carotid Artery

The term "carotid" comes from the Greek "karos" which means deep sleep. These vessels were so named by Galen, a Roman physician in the second century, A.D. because compressing them caused loss of consciousness. There are two of these arteries, one on each side of the front of the neck. They both extend upward to divide near the angle of the jaw into the internal and external carotid arteries. The internal carotid artery continues upward to pass through an opening in the base of the skull to supply the front and middle parts of the brain on its side. The external carotid artery continues upward outside the skull to supply the face, mouth, ear, and scalp.

Common Femoral Artery

The artery in the groin that supplies red blood to the entire leg.

Common Iliac Artery

The abdominal aorta divides at the level of the navel into two large vessels, each about three inches long, called the right and left common iliac arteries, respectively. Both divide into two vessels. One, called the *internal iliac artery,* supplies red blood to its half of the pelvis. The other, called the *external iliac artery,* supplies red blood to the leg below.

Coronary Arteries

The arteries that supply red blood to the heart muscle and enable the right ventricle to pump the blue blood to the lungs and the left ventricle to pump the red blood to the body. There are two of these vessels, a right and a left, and both arise from the base of the aorta. They are the first branches of the aorta. These two arteries, and their network of branches spread over the heart like a crown ("corona"), hence their name -- *coronaries.*

Coronary Bypass Surgery

Surgery that involves joining grafts that convey arterial (red) blood from an artery outside the heart to the open coronary arteries beyond sites of obstruction in these vessels. This new supply of red blood bypasses the sites of blockage and supplies oxygen, water, nutrients, and other chemicals to the tissues that had been deprived.

Superficial veins taken from the legs are frequently used as coronary artery bypass grafts (CABG's). These grafts are joined on one end to openings made in the body's biggest artery (the ascending aorta) and on the other end to openings made in the coronary arteries beyond the sites of blockage.

Small arteries can also be used as CABG's. The most common of these are the two *internal mammary arteries* that run one on each side of the sternum (breastbone). The upper end of a mammary graft is usually left attached to the artery going to the arm from which it arises. The lower end of the mammary artery graft is joined to an opening made in a coronary artery beyond the site of obstruction.

Coronary Heart Disease Due to Atherosclerosis

A condition in which there is an insufficient supply of oxygenated (red) blood to the heart muscle because the coronary arteries have become blocked as a result of hardening of their walls and clot formation on their flow surfaces (coronary thrombosis). This clotting occurs most often as a consequence of rupture of the lipid core of soft plaques which releases the fatty contents into the lumen and causes the blood to jell (clot) -- see Fig. 33, p. 74.

Coronary thrombosis also occurs from platelet aggregation and fibrin formation on rough and irregular atherosclerotic surfaces that have lost their covering of endothelial cells -- see Fig. 34, p. 75.

Patients with coronary disease often experience pain in the left side of the front of their chest with exercise or emotion. If thrombosis (clotting) occurs, the person may "drop dead."

Embolus
An object that breaks loose from the heart or vessel wall -- such as a fragment of a platelet aggregate, a portion of a clot, or a particle of an atherosclerotic deposit -- and is carried by the blood until it reaches a vessel that is too small for the embolus to pass through. The embolus plugs the vessel at that point and blocks the flow of blood to the tissues.

Endovascular Surgery
A recent surgical specialty that differs from open vascular surgery in the way the surgeon reaches the diseased vessel. The endovascular surgeon reaches the diseased artery through the flow channel, while in open vascular surgery the surgeon makes incisions and exposes the arteries from the outside. Then, the vascular surgeon either places a graft to bypass a blockage, opens the vessel and removes the obstruction, or places a graft to repair an aneurysm.

In endovascular surgery, the surgeon approaches the obstructed artery from the inside, i.e., through the flow channel, with catheters (long, slender, hollow tubes) to which devices attached to their distal ends (inflatable balloons, cutting instruments, or grinding burrs) are used to remove obstructions that block the flow channel.

The endovascular surgeon passes these catheters over guide wires into arteries that are usually far away from the sites of the obstructions to be treated. This new type of surgeon,with the guidance of continuous x-ray visualization, advances the guide wires, catheters, and operating devices to the proper location, as in the coronary arteries, and performs the endovascular operation.

Fats (Triglycerides)
Molecules that consist of three fatty acids chemically linked to an alcohol called glycerol. All fats contain mixtures of different types of fatty acids. Fatty acids consist of linear chains of carbon atoms with hydrogen atoms bound to them. Ninety-five percent of the fat stored in the fat cells of the adipose tissue is in the triglyceride form.

Fats may be classified as saturated or unsaturated. A saturated fatty acid has no double carbon=carbon bonds; all of the bonding sites are filled with hydrogen atoms. Unsaturated fatty acids contain one or more double carbon=carbon bonds. If a fatty acid has only one double bond, it is called monounsaturated. If it has two or more, it is polyunsaturated.

Saturated fats are solid at room temperature; unsaturated fats (oils) are liquid at room temperature. Both are insoluble in water. The body uses many fatty acids and can make all but two, linolenic and linoleic, which are polyunsaturated and must be in our diet.

Both olive and canola oils are examples of monounsaturated fats. These fats are protective against atherosclerosis. In addition, the polyunsaturated oils such as those in soybeans, corn, and safflower seeds are protective, too. Also, the polyunsaturated oils in fish, like salmon, tuna, trout, halibut, herring, and sardines, are also protective, possibly because they contain fatty acids which tend to prevent unwanted blood clotting.

Diets high in saturated fats and *trans* fatty acids are associated
with high blood levels of low density lipoprotein cholesterol
(LDL). This is so because the liver converts saturated fats and
trans fatty acids into LDL cholesterol. High blood levels of
this form of cholesterol are associated with the development of
atherosclerosis.

Prime sources of saturated fats are fatty meats, poultry skin
with attached fat, whole milk, butter, cream, ice cream,
candies, cakes, cheeses, and pastries.

Prime sources of *trans* fatty acids are hydrogenated or partially
hydrogenated polyunsaturated vegetable oils, such as the
soybean oil used in margarines, especially the hard types, and
products such as many cookies, crackers, cakes, candies,
doughnuts, and pastries made with any hydrogenated or
partially hydrogenated oils. Beware if the content label reads
"hydrogenated" to any degree.

Phospholipids are a type of fat that contains phosphorus. These
substances are the main components of the retaining walls,
both external and internal, of all our body's cells. These
membranes must be insoluble in water or they would quickly
dissolve. If our cell membranes were to suddenly dissolve, we
would die in seconds. From this aspect alone (and there are
many others), fat is an essential part of our diet. But, we must
severely restrict the saturated and *trans* fatty acid types. While
the mono and polyunsaturated types are protective of our
blood vessels, they are such a rich source of calories that they
should be taken in moderation.

Fiber
The portion of plant foods that our bodies can't digest. There
are two basic types of fiber -- soluble and insoluble. Insoluble
fiber helps the digestive system run smoothly and prevents
constipation. Soluble fiber decreases the absorption of

cholesterol by the bowel.

Insoluble fiber, referred to as "roughage," includes the woody part of plants, such as the skins of fruits and vegetables and the outer coating of grain and rice kernels.

Soluble fiber dissolves and thickens in water to form gels. Beans, barley, broccoli, citrus fruits, oatmeal, and especially oat bran are rich sources of soluble fiber.

Fiber is found only in complex carbohydrates. Whether soluble or insoluble, complex carbohydrates when coated by their protective fiber components are digested and absorbed more slowly than when the fiber has been removed by refining processes. For this reason, high-fiber complex carbohydrates decrease the sugar load on the islet cells of the pancreas and reduce the insulin response.

This is why the majority of our carbohydrate calories should come from high-fiber sources such as whole grain cereals, breads, and pastas; brown rice; fresh fruit; fresh vegetables; and legumes (peas, beans, and lentils).

This is also why we should restrict the calories we get from processed complex carbohydrates (such as white bread, mashed potatoes, french fries -- also have too much fat -- and white rice), because they have lost most of their fiber.

Sugar, a nonfiber carbohydrate, should be drastically restricted. The sugar we eat is mainly sucrose, a disaccharide ($C_{12}H_{22}O_{11}$), that is quickly combined in the bowel with water and converted into glucose, a monosaccharide ($C_6H_{12}O_6$), which is rapidly absorbed into the blood.

Fiber is also valuable because it contains many minerals, phytochemicals (plant chemicals), and vitamins.

Fibrin
An elastic, thread-like protein which is formed from fibrinogen, a protein in the blood. Fibrin molecules join together to form an insoluble compound that forms the essential portion or backbone of a blood clot.

Heart Attack
A condition in which part of the heart wall dies because of lack of blood supply, most often from obstruction (occlusion) of a coronary artery due to atherosclerosis and clot formation (thrombosis). The impact of the heart attack may be mild, moderate, severe, or even fatal depending on how much and which part of the heart muscle has lost its blood supply. The patient having a heart attack will often experience severe chest pain, become nauseated, sweat profusely, be short of breath, and have low blood pressure.

Hemoglobin
The iron containing protein in the red cells of our blood which combines with oxygen in the lungs to form a bright red compound called *oxyhemoglobin*. The red blood cells carry the oxyhemoglobin to the tissues where it supplies oxygen to the cells so they can live. After giving up oxygen, hemoglobin becomes a dark burgundy color and is called *reduced hemoglobin*. The more oxygen the blood gives up, the darker (more blackish) it becomes.

The change in color of hemoglobin in the pulmonary capillaries causes the blood in the pulmonary veins and systemic arteries to be bright red, and the change in the color of hemoglobin in the systemic capillaries causes the blood in our systemic veins and pulmonary arteries to be dark burgundy in color. Though not strictly accurate, venous blood is referred to as "blue."

Hemorrhage (Bleeding)
Loss of blood from a blood vessel. In external hemorrhage, the blood escapes from the body. In internal hemorrhage, the bleeding occurs into a body cavity or into the tissues surrounding the bleeding vessel.

High Blood Pressure (Hypertension)
Persistent or intermittent elevation of the blood pressure above the upper range of normal (140/90). Uncontrolled, chronic high blood pressure strains the heart; damages arteries; and creates a greater risk of heart attack, heart failure, stroke, kidney failure, and blindness.

Infarct
Refers to an area of tissue that has died as a result of lack of blood supply. A "myocardial infarct" is an area of dead heart muscle due to the blockage of its blood flow by obstruction of the coronary artery which supplied it.

Intermittent Claudication
Cramping pain that develops after variable degrees of exercise in muscles of the extremities due to an insufficient supply of arterial (red) blood. The most common muscles to be affected are those of the calf. The more restricted the blood supply, the shorter the distance a person can walk before cramping pain in the deprived muscles forces the individual to stop and rest. Claudication pain is intermittent because it is brought on by exercise and relieved by rest. The most common cause of intermittent claudication is the obstructive form of atherosclerosis.

The resting muscle has an adequate supply of red blood for its needs and is not painful. But the working muscle develops an inadequate blood supply because the obstructed artery that supplies it can't deliver enough blood during exercise. This inadequate blood supply causes the buildup of lactic acid in the tissues which produces pain. "Claudication" comes from the Latin and means "lameness."

Ischemia
A condition in which there is either an insufficient supply of arterial (red) blood to some part of the body due to obstruction of the artery supplying it and/or an inadequate output of blood by the heart.

Life Style
An individual's typical way of life, including home environment, diet, occupation, recreational pursuits, exercise routines, and smoking, drinking, and sleeping habits.

Lumen (channel)
The passageway inside a tubular organ. The vascular lumen is the passage for blood inside the walls of a blood vessel.

Metabolism
A general term designating all chemical changes which occur in the body.

Murmur
The sound generated by blood swirling within the heart or arteries. This turbulence occurs in the blood as it jets from a narrow channel into a large one.

Occlusion of a Blood Vessel
The closing or shutting off of a blood vessel's lumen (flow channel).

Open-Heart Surgery
Surgery performed on the opened heart under direct vision.

Peripheral Vascular Disease
A term which, in its broadest sense, refers to diseases of any of the blood vessels outside of the heart and to diseases of the lymph vessels.

Plaque
An atherosclerotic formation in the inner portion of the wall of an artery caused by infiltration of LDL cholesterol and fats. The plaque may be hard if much calcium is deposited in or around it, or soft if little is deposited. Soft plaques often develop a lipid core which can rupture and cause the blood to clot.

Plasma
The cell-free liquid portion of uncoagulated blood; serum is the liquid that remains after blood clots.

Platelets
One of the three kinds of formed elements found in the blood. The other two types are the red and white blood cells. Platelets don't have a nucleus; white cells do; circulating red cells do not.

Platelets initiate clot formation in the arterial system by forming aggregates. Also, platelets contain many growth factors that promote the healing of wounds.

Platelets are tiny pinched off portions of a large cell in the bone marrow called a *megakaryocyte*. These fragments float along in the outer portion of the blood stream ever ready should injury strike to initiate formation of a clot to plug up a hole in the vessel wall.

Platelets can also be triggered to cause clots by the fatty liquid that escapes from the lipid core of a ruptured soft plaque and by the abnormal flow surface of the diseased wall of a hardened artery. Such clots can kill us if they close off a vital vessel, as a coronary artery, and cause a fatal heart attack. Too few platelets can cause us to bleed to death. Too many can cause us to clot to death.

Platelets survive about 10 days after they are released into the blood from the bone marrow. Each second about 1-1/2 million platelets wear out and are replaced by 1-1/2 million new ones.

Proteins
Complex, big molecules constructed of long, three-dimensionally wrapped chains of combinations of amino acids. Amino acids are molecules constructed of four chemical units joined to a single carbon atom: an amino (NH_2) group, a hydrogen atom (H), a carboxylic acid (COOH) group, and a side-group containing various combinations of carbon, hydrogen, nitrogen (N), and sometimes sulfur (S). It is the side-groups that distinguish the 20 different amino acids that our bodies must have.

Of these 20 amino acids, nine can't be manufactured by our bodies and must be derived from the foods we eat. These amino acids, which we must have but can't manufacture, are called *essential* amino acids.

The body manufactures thousands of different types of proteins with these 20 amino acids. Each of these proteins has a single function. This function is determined by the order and shape of its amino acid chains.

Many vital structures inside our cells are made from proteins. For example, the ribosomes that make proteins, and the mitochondria that make energy are constructed with protein components. The enzymes that control the chemistry of our bodies are also proteins. The hemoglobin in our red blood cells that carries the oxygen upon which our lives depend is a protein. Our muscles are proteins. The eyes, ears, nose, skin, hair and other surface features of a person are constructed of proteins.

Clearly, proteins are essential for life. They are best obtained from fish, skinless poultry, eggs, milk, cheese, peas, beans, lentils, nuts, seeds and lean meat.

Pulse
The expansion of an artery which can be palpated with a finger when the heart contracts (systole) and pumps blood out into the aorta and its branches.

Risk Factors
Conditions that predispose to the development of a certain disease. For example, the following habits and conditions are risk factors for having a heart attack:
- Smoking.
- Eating a low-fiber diet high in saturated fats, *trans* fatty acids, sugar, and calories.
- Leading a sedentary life.
- Carrying significant excess weight (fat).
- Experiencing marked stress.
- Having a family history of heart disease.
- Possessing sticky platelets, high fibrinogen, low HDL cholesterol, high triglycerides, high LDL cholesterol, and/or elevated levels of homocysteine.
- Having high blood pressure, diabetes, gout, and/or low thyroid function.

Saphenous Vein

The greater saphenous vein, the longest vein in the body, runs just beneath the skin along the inside of the leg from ankle to groin where it then goes deep to join the big vein at that level. The patient's own saphenous veins are the most frequently used grafts to bypass obstructions of the coronary and leg arteries.

Sclerosis

Means "hardening," as in the term "atherosclerosis" and indicates that the wall of the artery has became hard.

Trans Fatty Acids (see Fats, page 273-274).

Hydrogenation of polyunsaturated vegetable oils converts them into the equivalent of saturated fats, as it does to the soybean oil in margarines.

Veins

The vessels that carry blood back to the heart. The systemic veins convey the deoxygenated (blue) blood from the body to the right side of the heart. The pulmonary veins convey the freshly oxygenated (red) blood from the lungs to the left side of the heart.

Veins have much thinner walls than arteries and don't develop the changes of atherosclerosis. But like arteries, their walls also have three layers (intima -- inner portion, media -- middle portion, and adventitia -- outer portion).

Index

Aneurysms, 5,72,77,82,83,108-111,195,197,201,240,241,263

AIDS, 66

Alveolus, 27

Angina Pectoris, 90,263

Angioplasty, 93,198-203
    Abdomen, 202,203,225,227,232,
    Carotid (brain), 221
    Coronary (heart), 198-203,206,207,209
    Legs, 202,203,225-227,232,235
    Renal (kidney), 222,223

Antibodies, 24

Anticoagulant, 263

Antioxidant Vitamins, 189

Aorta, 5,58,108,263

Aortogram, 110,264

Arrhythmia, 264

Arteries, 7,21,56,57,264

Arteriogram (Angiograms), 99,100,105-107

Aspirin, 190

Atherosclerosis, 4-6,72-79,82,83,87,111,115,116,264,265

Automatic Internal Cardiac Defibrillator (AICD), 253-255

Better Life Diet, 136-151,185-187

Bile, 28

Blocked Arteries, 4-6,72-81,88-107, *see* bypass grafts, angioplasty, and
    stents

Blood, 64-67

Blood Clotting, 68-70,72-80

Blood Pressure, 102,103,265

Body Systems, 16-39
    Cardiovascular (heart, vessels, and blood), 20,21,44-83
    Digestive, 28,29
    Endocrine, 34,35
    Hematopoetic (blood cell forming), 22,23
    Integumentary (skin), 38,39
    Lymphatic/Immune, 24,25
    Musculoskeletal, 18
    Nervous, 19
    Reproductive, 36,37
    Respiratory, 26,27
    Urinary, 30-33

Boundary Organ Concept, 40-43
Bypass Grafts, 196,208,210-219,224,228-231,236-239
Cancer, 24,25,66,116-118,123,141
Capillaries, 11,59,266
Carbohydrates, 40,136,137,139,140,142,266,275
Carbon Dioxide, 267
Cardiac Arrest and Ventricular Fibrillation, 250-252,267
Cardiologist, 90-93,268
Cardiopulmonary Resuscitation (CPR), 250-252,268
CAT Scan, 110,111
Catheter, 92, 273
Causes of Death, 5
Cell, 8-11
Cerebral Vascular Accident (Stroke -- Brain Attack), 94-101,268
Chlamydia Pneumoniae, 265
Cholesterol, 72,73,188,269
Collateral Circulation, 80,81,226,234,269,270
Collateral Vessels, 80,81,226,234,269,270
Common Carotid Artery, 94,95,270
Common Femoral Artery, 225-231,233,236-239,270
Common Iliac Artery, 108,232,270
Coronary Arteries, 52,53,271
Coronary Arteriograms, 86,92,93
Coronary Bypass Surgery, 204,205,208,210-215,218,219,271
Coronary Heart Disease, 74,75,88 93,272
Coronary Thrombosis, 272
CPR (Cardiopulmonary Resuscitation), 250-252,268
Diabetes, 34,137,143,146
Diagnosis of Aneurysms, 82,83,108-111
Diagnosis of Blocked Arteries, 88-107
    Brain, 94-101
    Heart, 88-93
    Kidney, 102,103
    Legs, 104-107
Dialysis, 32,33
    Hemodialysis, 32,33
    Peritoneal Dialysis, 33
Diastole, 50
Diet, 113-115,136-151,182-187
Dietary Goals, 140
Duplex (Doppler) Studies, 100,101
Echocardiogram, 90,91

Electrocardiogram, 85,246
Embolus, 70,71,94,96,98,272
Emphysema, 116,118,123,141
Endarterectomy, 195,196,221,233
Endothelium, 56-60
Endovascular Surgery, 194,198-203, 272,273 (also see angioplasty)
ERT (Estrogen replacement therapy), 88, 191
Exercise, 113-115,152-179,184-186
Fats (Triglycerides), 40,72,73,136-140,142,147-150,269,273,274
    Monounsaturated, 273,274
    Polyunsaturated, 273,274
    Saturated, 269,273,274
Fiber, 72,136,137,140,274,275
Fibrin, 69,276
Fibrinogen, 69,115,120,186,188,276
Food Guide Diagram, 142-144
Free Oxygen Radicals, 120,189
Gangrene, 105
Gene Therapy, 234
Glossary, 263-282
Granulocytes (White Blood Cells), 64-67
HDL Cholesterol, 72,73,115,188,269
Heart Attack, 88,89,276
Heart Failure, 54,55
Heart Healthy Living, 182-191
    Five Cardinal Rules, 184-187
    Simplified Program, 182-191
    Three Additional Strategies, 188-191
Heart Scan, 86,90
Heart Transplantation, 256-258
Heart Valve Repair or Replacement, 216-219
Hemoglobin, 46,47,120,276
Hemorrhage, 94,277
High Blood Pressure, 115,277
HIV, 66
Homocysteine, 72,115,186,188,189,191
Infarct, 277
Inflammation, 65
Insulin, 34, 137,146,150,151,266
Intermittent Claudication, 104,277,278
Internal Mammary Artery, 205,208,211,214,215,218
Ischemia, 278

LDL Cholesterol, 72,73,115,188,269
Life Cycle, 12-15
Life Style, 115,278
Liver, 28-29
Lose Excess Weight, 113,115,145,147-151
Lumen, 278
Lymphocytes, 65,66
Macrophages, 67
Magnesium, 191
Metabolism, 278
Monocytes, 67
MRI, 110
Murmur, 97,279
Myocardial Infarction, 88,89,277
Nutrition, 113-115,136-151,182,187
Ornish diet, 137,146,149,185,191
Osteoporosis, 154, 165
Open-Heart Surgery, 208,210-219,279
Pacemakers, Artificial for the Heart, 246-249
Pacemaking and Conduction Systems of the Heart, 243-245
Peripheral Vascular Disease, 279
Plaque, 279
    Hard, 4,73,75,264,265,279
    Lipid Core, 5,73,74,264,265,279
    Soft, 4,5,73,74,264,265,279
Plasma, 279
Platelet Aggregation, 67-71,190,279-280
Platelets, 22,23,64,65,67-71,279,280
Prayer of Saint Francis, 262
Prevention of Atherosclerosis, 76,112-191
    Dietary Information, 113-115,136-151,184-187
    Exercise, 115,152-179,184-186
    Smoking, 113-135,184-186
    Stress, 113-115,180,181,184-186
    Weight, 113-115,142-151
Pritikin diet, 137,146,149,185,191
Proteins, 40,136,137,140,142,269,280,281
PTCA, 200,202,206,207,209
Red Blood Cells, 64,65
Renin, 86,102,103
Research and Commitment, 281-294
Rest Pain, 104,105

Risk Factors for Heart Attack, 115,281
Salt, 191
Saphenous Vein, 205,210,212-214,219,237-239,281,282
SIDS, 116
Simplified Program for Heart-Healthy Living, 182-191
Sinus Node, 243,244
Smoking, 113-136,184-186
Spiritual Reflections, 259-262
Stents, 200,201,203-205,207,209,222,223,225,226,232,235
Stethoscope, 86,97
Stress, 113-115,180,181
Sugar, 72,136,137,139,140,145,150,151,186,266,267,269,275,276
Surgery to Increase the Blood Supply, 192-233,235-239
    to the Brain, 220,221
    to the Heart, 204-219
    to the Kidneys, 222-224
    to the Legs, 225-233,235-239
Surgical Procedures, 192-233,235-241,247,249,254,257
    Endovascular, 192,193,198-203,206,207,209,223,232,235
    Vascular, 192-197,208,210-215,218,219,221,224,228-231,233,
        236-241
Systole, 51
TIA, 71,94-101
Trans Fatty Acids, 72,115,136-140,273,274,282
Transplantation - Heart, 256-258
Transplantation - Kidney, 31-33
Treadmill, 90-32
Triglycerides (Fats), 41,72,136-140,145,147-150,188,273,274
Turbulence, 97
Two Main Complications of Atherosclerosis, 4-6,72-83
Ultrasound Studies, 86,100-102,110
    Aorta, 110
    Carotid,100,101
    Kidneys, 102
    Legs, 86
Valves of Heart, 48-49
Valves of Veins, 60,62,63
Vascular Surgery, 194-197 (also see Surgical Procedures, Vascular)
Veins, 60-63,282
Weight - Loss of excess, 113-115,145,147-151
White Blood Cells (Granulocytes), 64-67

Review Questions to Help You
Help Others Beat Heart Disease
(Answers found on pages as listed)

1. If you were God, how would you build the human body? **1-308.**

2. What is the boundary organ concept? **40-43**

3. What are the three main parts of the cardiovascular system? **20**

4. What makes the blood in systemic arteries red and the blood in systemic veins blue? **46,47,276,277**

5. What do platelets and fibrinogen have to do with blood clotting? **67-71**

6. Are "hardening of the arteries" and "atherosclerosis" the same thing? **72**

7. Is it true that hardening of the arteries and clot formation kill more people in the United States than cancer, accidents, and infections combined? **5**

8. What are the two main complications of atherosclerosis? **77**

9. Where do arterial blockages occur most commonly? **87**

10. Where do aneurysms develop most often? **108**

11. What is "angina?" **90**

12. What are hard and soft plaques? **73-75**

13. What is a "heart attack?" **88,89,276**

14. What is the most common cause of heart attacks? **73-75**

15. What are the signs of a heart attack (**89**), a TIA (**98**), a stroke (**95**), a kidney that lacks an adequate blood supply (**102**), and of a leg that doesn't have enough blood supply (**104-107**)?

16. If 90% of deaths from premature cardiovascular disease can be prevented, why don't we do it? **113,114**

17. Why do smokers die an average of six to eight years sooner than nonsmokers? **116**

18. What is a "carbohydrate" (**266,267**), a "fat" (**273,275**), and a "protein?" (**280,281**)?

19. What is the difference between HDL cholesterol and LDL cholesterol? **73,269**

20. Why should saturated fats and *trans* fatty acids be severely restricted? **136,269,273,274**

21. Why should refined sugar be severely restricted? **136,137,145,147**

22. What is "fiber?" **274,275**

23. Why are high-fiber carbohydrates good for you but low-fiber carbohydrates are not? **137,275,276**

24. Where does 90% of the salt in our diet come from? **191**

25. How does a diet high in sugar and high in low-fiber complex carbohydrates cause diabetes? **137,147**

26. What's wrong with the "Standard American Diet?" **136**

27. What are the goals of The Better Life Diet? **140**

28. Who should follow The Better Life Diet? **136,137**

29. Who should follow the Pritikin or Ornish diets? **136,137,191**

30. What must one do to successfully lose excess fat, add muscle and then maintain the desired weight? **150,151**

31. Why is aerobic exercise essential for health? **152-155**

32. Is the simple "talk test" all you need to find the aerobic exercise pace that's right for you? **156-157**

33. What makes walking such a good exercise for nearly everyone? **166-167**

34. What are the five cardinal rules for heart-healthy living? **184-186**

35. What do the letters -- S ... D-E-W ... S -- help you remember? **184-186**

36. What are the two general types of operations for arterial disease? **194**

37. How is endovascular surgery performed? **198-199**

38. What is a "CABG?" **271**

39. What is a "PTCA?" **200**

40. How does an artificial pacemaker for the heart work? **246-249**

41. How should "CPR" be performed? **250-252**

42. Whom do you call when a heart emergency occurs and what information do you give? **250-252**

43. What is an AICD? **253-255**

44. Why were there only 2,500 heart transplants done in the United States last year? **256**

45. How to find increased happiness in your life. **259-262**

Need for Research

When I founded **The Hope Heart Institute** in 1959 there was a pressing need to develop better operations and means with which to treat patients afflicted with heart and blood vessel diseases. During the next 25 years the Institute developed an international reputation as my staff and I made many important discoveries, including development of:

1. The coronary bypass operation using the patient's own veins in 1962.
2. Improved artificial grafts to replace or bypass diseased arteries during the 1970's.
3. Operations to bring blood to the *entire* heart using *only* the internal mammary arteries in 1984.

In the 1980's the Institute broadened its research scope to include prevention as well as treatment of heart disease. These new studies proved successful and pointed the way for future work designed to decrease the need for surgery.

During this same period the Institute developed a major educational mission for the lay public through creation of the **Hope Health Letter**, a monthly publication designed to help healthy people stay healthy. Today six million people read each issue and millions more read other materials written by the educational staff under the direction of Carol Garzona.

The 1990's have been a time of intense investigative excitement at the Institute as its dedicated scientific staff has identified key research questions facing the field of cardiovascular disease and has accepted the challenge of contributing to their solutions. To aid in this effort, departments of Molecular Biology, Medical Engineering, and Clinical Research have been added to those established in earlier years -- Chemistry and Hematology, Surgery, Cell Biology, Histology, and Vascular Healing.

The recent discovery by the Institute's staff that there is a healing cell in the blood which can convert the inner surface of an artificial blood vessel graft into a living natural structure is of the utmost importance. The Institute is committed to learning where this cell originates and determining how to control and extend its healing potential.

Such basic scientific information could be of enormous biologic importance because it would:
1. Advance understanding of how blood cells form and blood vessels develop and heal.
2. Direct how to design better artificial blood vessels.
3. Identify ways to deploy this healing cell to rapidly heal such grafts in the coronary arteries of the heart and in the small arteries below the knees.
4. Add knowledge to help prevent hardening of the arteries (the cause of 95% of heart disease).
5. Provide new insights as to how to stop tumors from developing the blood supply they need to grow, spread, and kill their victims.

The possibilities for these major advances are real and must be pursued with full intensity because more people still die of heart and artery diseases than die of cancer, accidents, and infections combined.

The Hope Heart Institute faces the future with optimism based on past discoveries, current research, and on a passionate belief that diseases due to hardening of the arteries and clot formation can be defeated.

Though we are still far from victory in this all-out struggle for humankind, I believe that heart and artery disease as we know it today can be overcome in our time. I see this book as a force to empower people to help themselves and in turn to help others in this crucial struggle to defeat the Western world's greatest killers.

My goal in writing this book has been to help people live longer, healthier, and happier lives. You have a vital role to play. I now ask you to take my words and turn them into your everyday actions. Please encourage your family and your friends to do the same. By working together we will **beat heart disease.**

To join the Hope Heart team, please call or write:

The Hope Heart Institute
528 18th Avenue
Seattle, WA 98122
Phone: (206) 320-2001
Fax: (206) 323-2300

The Institute has outgrown its facilities and space, and must have a new research building, which will cost about $20 million. Your kind help would further the goal of eradicating heart disease. If possible, please send your tax-exempt gift labeled "Building Fund" to the above address.

Thank you for your generosity.

Sincerely,

Lester R. Sauvage, MD
Founder, The Hope Heart Institute

About the Author

LESTER R. SAUVAGE, M.D., author and world-renowned heart surgeon and research scientist, is clinical professor of surgery emeritus at the University of Washington and Founder of The Hope Heart Institute in Seattle where he is also Medical Director Emeritus. He has authored 235 articles on heart and blood vessel research and surgery, a monograph on heart valve replacement, and recently, an acclaimed inspirational book, *The Open Heart:Updated Edition.* In addition, he pioneered the first experimental coronary bypass surgery using veins, and the first use of the internal thoracic arteries to revascularize the entire human heart. Also, he pioneered the development of a line of artifical arteries, known as the *Sauvage Graft,* that are used world-wide.

Dr. Sauvage is certified by the American Board of Surgery and the American Board of Thoracic Surgery. He has also been awarded certificates for special competence in the surgery of infants and children and in vascular surgery.

His many honors and awards include:
• Alpha Omega Alpha National Honorary Medical Society, 1947.
• Member, Alpha Sigma Nu National Jesuit Honor Society, 1948.
• The degree HONORIS CAUSA, Seattle University, 1976.
• The Brotherhood Award, National Conference of
  Christians and Jews, 1979.
• The Clemson Award, Clemson University, for outstanding contributions
  in applied research on biomaterials, 1982.
• The degree of Doctor of Science, Gonzaga University, 1982.
• The Jefferson Award, American Institute for Public Service, 1983.
• The Governor's (Washington State) Distinguished
  Volunteer Award, 1983.
• The Washington State Medal of Merit, 1987.
• Honorary member of the New England Vascular Society, 1987.
• Seattle First Citizen Award, Seattle-King County
  Association of Realtors, 1992.
• Member, The American Surgical Association, 1995.
• Knight, The Equestrian Order of the Holy Sepulchre of Jerusalem, 1995.

About the Prevention Consultant

CAROL P. GARZONA, Director of Health Communications at The Hope Heart Institute and Editor of the **Hope Health Letter** and related products, received her undergraduate and graduate training in health communication theory and public health at the University of Washington. Carol's publications are read by millions of people each month.

About the Illustration Team

KATHRYN D. BARKER, Medical Artist and Calligrapher, received her undergraduate and graduate degrees in art from the University of Michigan. Kathryn has been actively working in the field of medical art for 20 years and is widely known for the beauty, clarity, and accuracy of her illustrations.

WARREN A. BERRY, Director of Computer Graphics and Medical Photography at The Hope Heart Institute, received his undergraduate training in multimedia production at the University of Washington and subsequently worked for many years at the School of Medicine in CCTV and later in commercial TV. His talent and drive have inspired each of us to "get our job done right."

A message from Better Life Press:

If you would like
Dr. Sauvage
to speak to your group on issues like:

- **How to experience happiness**

- **Understanding heart disease**

- **Living longer made easy**

- **Surgery should have a limited role**

Call Stan Emert at 206/323-0116, or via email at EmertStan1@aol.com. Dr. Sauvage has spoken to many associations, conventions, schools, business meetings, book clubs, and gatherings of many kinds. Dr. Sauvage accepts a limited number of speaking engagements each year to discuss hope, health and happiness, or, as he says, "The **How** and the **Why** to Live."

If you have any questions concerning bulk purchases of this book, its companion, *The Open Heart,* or any book from **Better Life Press**, please contact the publisher at 1104 Boren Avenue, Suite 323, Seattle, Washington, U.S.A. 98104. Phone: 206/323-0116; E-mail: SauvageBLP@aol.com.

If you are a book retailer or other book seller, please contact **Independent Publishers Group**, 814 N. Franklin Street, Chicago, Illinois, U.S.A. 60610. Phone: 800/888-4741 or 312/337-0747.

Endorsements
(Continued from front of book)

"In *You Can Beat Heart Disease,* Dr. Lester Sauvage, a renowned cardiovascular surgeon, describes in simple everyday language what the cardiovascular system is and how it works and relates to the rest of the body. Moreover, he clearly explains the disease process, hardening of the arteries, which can cause the breakdown of this vital system, the major cause of death in the United States. But above all, *You Can Beat Heart Disease* is a message of hope clearly pointing out successful treatment options for patients with cardiovascular disease while emphasizing a simple step-by-step program for the prevention of this scourge of modern civilization. Dr. Sauvage has produced a *real gem.*"

- John A. Mannick, MD
Mosely Distinguished Professor of Surgery
Harvard Medical School, Boston, Massachusetts

"You Can Beat Heart Disease gives the reader a step-by-step, highly effective plan for combating the *deadliest disease* in the industrialized world. If keeping your heart healthy concerns you, consider adding this authoritative, clearly written, and easily understood guide to your personal library."

- Denton A. Cooley, MD
President and Surgeon-in-Chief
Texas Heart Institute, Houston, Texas

"You Can Beat Heart Disease is an excellent overview of the cardiovascular system in language which both interests and informs and is *extremely readable.* The philosophy which Dr. Sauvage promotes is not only sensible and practical but properly emphasizes how our bodies can be made healthier and kept that way, and he rightly stresses the importance of our inner spiritual needs. The book deserves to bewidely accepted, and it should be compulsory reading for all medical, nursing, and related professionals."

- S. A. Mellick, CBE, MD
Vascular Surgeon, Brisbane, Australia
Past President (1991-93), International Society for Cardiovascular Surgery

"This outstanding book provides the essential knowledge you need to prevent and treat diseases of the heart and arteries. Dr. Sauvage communicates his powerful message in the same passionate manner that he taught me vascular surgery almost thirty years ago."

- **Yasutsugu Nakagawa, MD**
Director, Division of Cardiovascular Surgery
Chiba Cardiopulmonary Center, Chiba, Japan

"The authors have been able to put the most current information regarding the prevention and treatment of heart disease into proper perspective. This precise, easy-to-read, concise book with fast moving text and beautiful illustrations will dispel confusion and settle controversies for its fortunate readers. In the true sense of the word, this is a *self-help book for everyone.*"

- **Malay Patel, MD**
Vascular Surgeon, Ahmedabad, India

"This remarkable, small volume represents a precious distillate of Lester Sauvage's life-long experience with every aspect of the prevention and treatment of diseases of the heart and arteries. Importantly, this concisely written, well illustrated, and easily understood book is potentially a life saving aid for all of us and should be read by everyone."

- **Mr. Aires A.B. Barros D'Sa, MD**
Consultant Vascular Surgeon, Vascular Surgery Unit
Royal Victoria Hospital/The Queen's University, Belfast, United Kingdom

"This highly readable up-to-date description of heart and blood vessel problems and their management is a great book for professionals and non-professionals alike."

- **Robert L. Kistner, MD**
Straub Clinic & Hospital, Honolulu, Hawaii

"Maimonides, 1135-1204, believed that study of the marvels of the human body deepened one's faith in God. He further believed that the acquisition of medical skill and wisdom expanded one's intellectual capacity to recognize the awesome power of human and divine spirituality.

"Dr. Lester Sauvage has achieved all this and more in his very personal presentation of the human body with particular emphasis on the circulatory system. I enjoyed reading this book for many reasons and learned much from it that is ordinarily not appreciated. For example, I never realized how many and how fast red blood cells are recycled! This is a *terrific, easily readable book* that should be required reading by the general public."

- Herbert Dardik, MD
Clinical Professor of Surgery, Mount Sinai School of Medicine,
New York, New York
Chief of Vascular Surgery, Englewood Hospital and Medical Center,
Englewood, New Jersey

"This book by Dr. Sauvage and his staff focuses clearly on cardiovascular disease, the number one killer of Americans, and emphasizes what we need to know about its detection, management, and prevention. Those who carefully read Yo*u Can Beat Heart Disease* will make the lifestyle choices necessary to keep themselves healthy. Just imagine the positive impact on our health care system if we would all do this."

- Ronald J. Stoney, MD
Professor of Surgery Emeritus
University of California, San Francisco

"You Can Beat Heart Disease is succinct, highly readable, and authoritative. It should be invaluable to readers interested in the primary or secondary prevention of heart disease. Anyone with atherosclerosis will find this well organized text to be very useful, especially should they be considering a revascularization procedure, because well informed patients tend to have markedly better outcomes."

- Floyd D. Loop, MD
Chief Executive Officer
The Cleveland Clinic Foundation, Cleveland, Ohio

"You Can Beat Heart Disease is a unique book with the clear objective of helping to defeat heart disease by empowering the reader with easily understandable and highly useful information.   This book has been written specifically for the lay public and is *exceptionally well organized.* It begins with an overview of relevant biologic processes, progresses to specific clinical diseases, and then factually discusses the advantages and disadvantages of the prevention and treatment options that are available. Because this book has the information I want my patients and their families to have, I will strongly recommend it to them."

- Howard P. Greisler, MD
Professor of Surgery
Division of Vascular Surgery
Loyola University Medical Center, Maywood, Illinois

"I found Lester Sauvage's new book, *You Can Beat Heart Disease,* to be extremely informative and highly useful -- likely the best in its class. I will order it to be distributed to my patients."

- Francis Robicsek, MD, PhD
Chairman, Department of Thoracic and Cardiovascular Surgery
Carolinas Medical Center, Charlotte, North Carolina
Clinical Professor of Surgery, University of North Carolina

"This book is about much more than heart disease, it is a *prescription for good health*, and describes in clear terms how to use this knowledge."

- Malcolm O. Perry, MD
Chairman of Surgery, St. Paul Medical Center, Dallas, Texas

"Lester Sauvage has brought us an invaluable compendium of heart information in a manner we can all understand. This book is a *must for all -- sick or well."*

- Lloyd M. Nyhus, MD
Professor of Surgery, Emeritus
University of Illinois, Chicago

"*I read every page* of this compact volume and found it to be most informative. I predict that it will be very helpful to lay individuals -- and to doctors as well!"

- **Jesse E. Thompson, MD, FACS**
Vascular Surgeon and Director Emeritus, Division of Vascular Surgery
Baylor University Medical Center, Dallas, Texas
Past President (1983-85), International Society for Cardiovascular Surgery

"This is a much-needed book to help the public understand cardiovascular disease, the number one killer in the United States. The book contains up-to-date and easy-to-read information about the mechanisms of the disease processes, the diagnosis, and most importantly, a clear explanation of the modern treatments for cardiovascular disorders."

- **James S.T. Yao, MD, PhD**
Magerstadt Professor of Surgery
Northwestern University Medical School, Chicago, Illinois

"Dr. Lester Sauvage and his team have succeeded in the *monumental task* of summarizing the great mound of information relating to atherosclerotic heart and artery disease into a relatively small volume of easily understood English prose suitable for reading by the lay public. My congratulations to them for undertaking this great and worthy task."

- **Anthony M. Imparato, MD**
Professor of Surgery
Division of Vascular Surgery
New York University Medical Center, New York, New York

"This book presents a clear and concise overview of cardiovascular disease: its causes, effects, treatment, and prevention. Written in a very readable format with good illustrations, this book will be very useful for patients and their families. It will also be valuable for those of us who wish to avoid the disastrous consequences of hardening of our arteries and clot formation."

- **Christopher K. Zarins, MD**
Chidester Professor of Surgery and Chief of Vascular Surgery,
Stanford University, Stanford, California

"I *enjoyed* reading *this book immensely* and firmly believe that an understanding of the physical and spiritual principles underlying the function of the body is essential for a healthy heart."

- Glenn C. Hunter, MD
Professor of Surgery, Section of Vascular Surgery
University of Texas Medical Branch, Galveston, Texas

"Pleasantly informative, scientifically accurate, well illustrated, and *written in grand style.*"

- John J. Bergan, MD
Professor of Surgery
Loma Linda University, Loma Linda, California
University of California, San Diego, California
Uniformed Services University of the Health Sciences, Bethesda, Maryland

"This book was *easy to read* and *easy to understand.* In my opinion, it is an *ideal book* about a *vital subject* that will, I am sure, benefit the general public, cardiovascular patients, and even their doctors."

- Charles Rob, MD
Professor of Surgery
Uniformed Services University of the Health Sciences, Bethesda, Maryland
Past President (1959-61), International Society for Cardiovascular Surgery

"This *concise book* addresses the risk factors associated with the development of heart and artery diseases and provides a detailed approach that will help you keep well. *You Can Beat Heart Disease* is important for potential patients (nearly everyone), actual patients, and physicians alike."

- Thomas J. Fogarty, MD
Professor of Surgery
Division of Vascular Surgery
Stanford University School of Medicine, Stanford, California

"Dr. Sauvage has had great experience in the surgical management of patients with heart disease. And he has now produced a book, *You Can Beat Heart Disease,* which, if followed, will clearly reduce the need for heart surgery. This book will be of particular value to those with increased risk factors for coronary artery disease."

- **John Ochsner, MD**
Chairman Emeritus, Dept of Surgery
Ochsner Clinic, New Orleans, Louisiana
Past President (1989-91), International Society for Cardiovascular Surgery

"Most other books in this field deal with a single factor -- for example, diet, exercise, smoking, weight, stress, or medications -- and describe how the action, absence, addition, and proper or improper use of this one factor will accelerate, slow down, prevent, or possibly even reverse the development of heart and artery disease. But experience has shown that correcting or modifying one factor is seldom effective in stopping heart disease.

"By contrast, Dr. Sauvage's new book tackles all of the many factors pertinent to the cause, prevention, and treatment of heart and artery disease in a single, concise volume. By doing so he illuminates why all these factors must be marshalled into one powerful force to defeat cardiovascular disease, the greatest killer in the United States.

"Now that I have a book that tells me how to live a long and healthy life in clear words I can easily understand, I will use it to help my family and friends as well as myself. *This book is a true message of life,* and it will be my routine gift from this time on."

- **John F. (Jack) Kiley**
Recent coronary bypass patient, Olympia, Washington

"Dr. Sauvage's new *book* is an owner's manual for the human heart. Packed with useful information and helpful illustrations, it strips the confusion and mystery from the prevention of heart disease. At long last, here *is* the *user-friendly* resource that belongs in every household."

- **Nicholas J. Bez**
Philanthropist, Seattle, Washington

"You Can Beat Heart Disease is a wonderful resource for heart patients and anyone interested in good health."
- **Joseph C. Piscatella**
Author, *Don't Eat Your Heart Out,* Tacoma, Washington

"I really enjoyed reading this book. I must admit I find that most books for the lay public fail to strike a good balance between simplicity and enough information. This book is unique because it strikes that balance. In doing this, it gives a good idea about the underlying biology and discusses therapeutic approaches in a fair way that should be very helpful to patients trying to understand their physician's instructions."

- **Stephen M. Schwartz, MD, PhD**
Professor of Pathology
University of Washington School of Medicine, Seattle, Washington

"This is a *wonderful book* for my patients."
- **J. Ward Kennedy, MD**
Robert A. Bruce Professor of Medicine
University of Washington School of Medicine, Seattle, Washington

"This *timely monograph* provides an excellent balance of information regarding heart disease with equal attention to basic pathophysiology, practical patient efforts, and sophisticated medical interventions. As such, it will elicit broad interest from those who wish a comprehensive yet clear introduction to the prevention and treatment of heart disease. *I highly recommend this book."*

- **Bradford C. Berk, MD, PhD**
Director of Cardiovascular Research
University of Washington School of Medicine, Seattle, Washington

"This book by a pioneer in the development of surgical techniques to treat heart disease is particularly valuable because it demonstrates how each of us can take control of our cardiovascular health status. Bravo, Dr. Sauvage!"

- **Kaj H. Johansen, MD, PhD**
Professor of Surgery, University of Washington School of Medicine
Seattle, Washington

"Dr. Sauvage and his collaborators have prepared an *unusually comprehensive basic* and factual treatise on the biology of the circulatory system with an emphasis on atherosclerosis and heart disease. Its engaging style and highly understandable language will make this concise book appealing to the vast audience of those who aren't schooled in the words of medicine. Many sections such as the one detailing the essentials of an excellent program to abandon smoking makes it an especially useful guide to develop a heart-healthy lifestyle.

"Also impressive is Dr. Sauvage's understanding and clear delineation of the importance that an attitude of faith and hope plays in one's well-being."

- **Vallee L. Willman, MD**
Professor and Chairman Emeritus
St. Louis University School of Medicine, St. Louis, Missouri

"You Can Beat Heart Disease is an *essential book* for patients, families of patients, and physicians who have anything to do with taking care of patients with coronary or peripheral arterial disease. This concise, well-written text explains in accurate but simple terms the concepts of heart and artery diseases that are often misinterpreted and misevaluated by patients and physicians alike.

"This book is *invaluable* because it lets the readers understand that they have as much control over their own destiny as the physicians taking care of them. It instructs the patients on how to extend their longevity by modifying how they live their lives. I wholeheartedly recommend this book to anyone who intends to live over 50 years in the American culture."

- **R. Clement Darling III, MD**
Associate Professor of Surgery
Albany Medical College, Albany, New York

"This book will help you beat heart disease."

- **John W. Kirklin, MD**
Professor of Surgery, Department of Surgery
University of Alabama at Birmingham

"Here is a collection of valuable, clearly presented, in-depth discussions about the causes, prevention, and treatment -- both medical and surgical -- of heart and artery diseases. Preventive measures are stressed, and the spiritual dimensions of life and service to others are unblushingly set out in this concise handbook."

- C. Rollins Hanlon, MD, FACS
Executive Consultant, Director General Emeritus
American College of Surgeons, Chicago, Illinois

"I have just finished your book, and I think it is outstanding. Congratulations! I hope it becomes a best seller.

"I particularly enjoyed the parts on smoking cessation, dietary management, exercise, and the control of stress. It really *covers all the topics extremely well and is very easy reading and enjoyable.* You have my total support for achieving maximal circulation of this important book. It will help many people, and I will use it for my patients."

- Frank J. Veith, MD
Professor & Chief of Vascular Surgical Services
Montefiore Medical Center &
Albert Einstein College of Medicine
New York, New York

"A *book* like this is *sorely needed,* so much so that I thought of doing one myself. Now that my good friend and colleague, Lester Sauvage, has done it so well, I can set this task aside. He has done us all a favor, and, as usual, *done it to perfection."*

- Robert B. Rutherford, MD
Emeritus Professor of Surgery
University of Colorado, Denver, Colorado

"Heart disease is *largely preventable*. In his book, *You Can Beat Heart Disease,* Dr. Sauvage and his team have clearly outlined the *principles* for us to *follow* to prolong our survival. **However, even a perfect lifestyle will not prevent the inevitable . . . we will all ultimately die.**

"Bodily well-being must not be our only goal. We also need to nourish and exercise our spiritual lives. We must decide what we believe about God, how we will relate to Him, and how our relationship with God will affect our interactions with others. That is why you must also read Dr. Sauvage's other book, *The Open Heart,* to complete the story. In it he describes how a life crisis can (and should) bring us closer to God. These two books, written by a surgeon who has held and healed many hearts, will help us to achieve both physical and spiritual health."

- **H. Leon Greene, MD**
Professor of Medicine, University of Washington
Author, *If I Should Wake Before I Die*
Seattle, Washington

"Besides being a skillful and caring surgeon, Dr. Sauvage is a talented writer. It is not common to see these two attributes together. His book *You Can Beat Heart Disease* is *concise, clear,* and *well organized.* Simple, but clear line drawings and half tone illustrations make it easy for the lay person to understand and enjoy the marvels of human biology, anatomy, and physiology.

"The most common diseases affecting the cardiovascular system are masterfully described in terms that everybody can understand. Their prevention and treatment are state of the art and a joy to read. Dr. Sauvage's book is full of common sense and sound advice that we must heed to live a quality life. A *fitting ending to this wonderful book is the Prayer of St. Francis.* The problems cursing our health care system today would be greatly lessened by remembering its closing words:

'For it is in giving that we receive,
it is in pardoning that we are pardoned,
and it is in dying
that we are born to eternal life.'"

- **J. Leonel Villavicencio, MD**
Professor of Surgery
Uniformed Services University of the Health Sciences, Bethesda, Maryland

Concluding Thoughts

Dr. H. Leon Greene says in his endorsement on the previous page, "You must also read Dr. Sauvage's other book, *The Open Heart,* to complete the story." The combination of *You Can Beat Heart Disease* and *The Open Heart* speaks to the twin goals of achieving a long, happy and healthy life here on earth, and then enjoying the infinitely greater joy of Heaven for all eternity. In brief, these goals are the essence of **the how and the why to live.**

Writing the "whole" story for you has been a passion that grew within my soul as I performed open-heart surgery for 33 years. Having time to write these books after retiring from operative surgery has been a source of great happiness to me.

In closing, I suggest that we can make the world a better place for all, at least to some degree, if we have the courage and the will to do so. We can do this by putting God's love into full action in our lives. In doing this we will become happier than we have ever been.

Why not? The time for this action is now. For the love of God and humankind, let's do it.

Sincerely,

Lester R. Sauvage, MD,
Founder,
The Hope Heart Institute
528 18th Avenue
Seattle, WA 98122